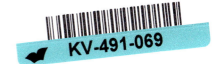

LIVE WELL BEYOND BREAST CANCER

How to Get through Treatment and Back to a Life You Love

BIRGITTE L. WILMS

ISBN: 978-19-5-315333-3

Published by

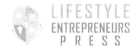

If you are interested in publishing through
Lifestyle Entrepreneurs Press, write to:
Publishing@LifestyleEntrepreneursPress.com

Publications or foreign rights acquisition of our catalog books.
Learn More: *www.LifestyleEntrepreneursPress.com*

Printed in the USA

Advance Praise

"I could not put this book down! Not only is the book very readable, it is full of information for those who struggle with breast cancer, and full of emotions and insights into the human psyche, all sprinkled with a little humor! The author's journey is unique but still relatable and inspirational. Often raw but full of positivity. I recommend this book to everyone with breast cancer and those who surround them."

—Laila Jonsson

"As someone with personal experience with breast cancer, I can honestly say this book should be required reading for anyone diagnosed with breast cancer, anyone who knows someone with breast cancer or anyone who may get it. Birgitte has succeeded in communicating the complex emotions, pain, despair, fear and ultimately her triumph in a powerful and meaningful way. There are lessons to be learned for anyone reading her saga from dealing with the initial diagnosis to the complexity of treatment options and all the associated feelings and difficulties. However, where this story really shines in the profound sense of hope she communicates about living life after cancer. After reading this, you will be inspired to find renewed beauty in life and in living life nor just surviving."

—Faith Ortins

"I didn't know what to expect reading Birgitte's book. I can't imagine being diagnosed with such an advanced stage of cancer. Now I know if I ever have the misfortune of being faced with breast cancer, I can turn to Birgitte's book for guidance and reassurance that I can get thru this and return to my best life ever. Thank you for your personal account and courage."

—Ginny Chiusano

"I would invite Cancer patients/survivors at any stage or years ago; please read this book, *Live Well beyond Breast Cancer*. It's a great story of a woman's journey that is inspirational to all.

It doesn't matter where you are in your journey. This read is so worth the investment in You, whether to gain healthy perspectives or validate what you already know. I was truly validated that albeit I was done with cancer and thought I'd never want to talk about breast cancer, yet here I feel I can embrace it now. I had it. It's gone but I'll always watch for it.

Live Well beyond Breast Cancer is a very easy relaxing book. The writer is so invested; authentic.

She writes short chapters. And, It's not all about cancer. It's about finding what works for you. She's grateful and so am I; that she wrote it down then made it available to all.

I call it authentic, succinct, and liberating. Ms. Wilms really gave me an emotional lifeline. I'm going to read it again. It only takes a couple hours."

—Julianne Ziefle

"Such a great and amazing book ! So real, touching and practical! Has everything you need to navigate the journey of cancer. I highly recommend it to everyone who is going through cancer. Great advice and so much to learn !"

—Jelena Spasovski

"Facing a sudden diagnosis of stage 3 Breast Cancer, having recently adopted her first child and in the beginning process of a second adoption there was only one direction to go. This is a well told story, a resource that is honest, supportive and a straight forward read for anyone. There is excellent life to be lived and the help and connections to let us live it...cancer be damned! *Live Well beyond Breast Cancer* is not a title that I would be drawn to. I am a voracious reader in many genres, including occasional self-development books - but I have never personally suffered serious illness so this would not be my normal pick. I was completely taken in.!!!

Using perfectly poignant quotes from others: "Hope and fear cannot occupy the same space at the same time. Invite one to stay."—Maya Angelou and creating quotable moments of her own:

"Once you take hold of an emotion it becomes our walking stick, something we won't let go of even if it doesn't benefit us in any way."

This is no Pollyanna story.

Birgitte L. Wilms does not sidestep significant issues and fears.

I found relief in her honesty sharing the whole experience including the elevated self and the depths that human suffering can bring."

—Annie Schneider

"*Live Well beyond Breast Cancer - How to Get Through Treatment and Back to a Life you Love* by Birgitte l. Wilms, is a wonderful and positive book. It takes a terrifying and potentially overwhelming topic and tackles it head on with an enlightening manner uplifting to the soul.

One will follow the writer's personal journey through her own harrowing experience but never feel mired down by a 'Pity Me' perspective. In fact, the author urges the reader to always focus on searching for gratitude in their own lives and seeking positivity to aid in their own personal healing while they battle through the fight of their lives.

I see this book on many waiting room tables in Oncology offices and Dr. offices. Ms. Wilms has covered easily from beginning to end the Breast Cancer process and this book would be helpful for those new to cancer or even for family members learning to understand what their loved ones are enduring. I urge everyone to read it. You will not be disappointed."

—Eden F. Lefebvre

"I just finished reading *Live Well beyond Breast Cancer*. An open and honest look at a journey from diagnosis through treatment and recovery. As a fellow cancer warrior, I understand how sharing stories can be supportive and this book does just that. I would highly recommend this book to a newly diagnosed patient or their family members to know you are not alone and you really can get back to a life you love."

—Heather Kulenski

"From the first sentence Birgitte makes clear that her message is aimed straight at women who are about to go through, or are already enduring, the ordeal that is breast cancer. But if that is not you, don't be too quick to set this book aside. This book could just as easily be called "Live Well Beyond Cancer" (of most any kind, I imagine), as there are valuable insights here for the many others who will inevitably be touched by the experience:

spouses, partners, friends, caregivers and family members. The narrative is grounded in very clearly expressed personal experience, so of course there is a huge amount of detail that is specific to breast cancer. Nevertheless, there is much here for anyone, female or male, who is going through an unexpected traumatic event. Birgitte has navigated her journey with courage and insight, and has come through whole. Perhaps this book can help you do the same."

—Pam Najera

"Birgitte graciously shares her personal journey with stage 4 breast cancer in order to show you that it is possible to get back to the life you love despite the rough speed bumps this cancer inevitably puts in your path. This book is not intended to be a medical tome replete with all the latest scientific discoveries and treatment options. Rather, grab a cup of green tea, (which Birgitte mixes with other flavored teas to improve the taste!), and sit down with an empathetic and companionable friend who is willing to share her personal experience factually and realistically with you to let you know that you are not alone on this journey. This book is about inspiring you to put yourself first, and to ask for, and accept, the support and love of friends and family who give us all the strength we need to persevere. There are tips, of course, on the need to eat a healthier diet, lower sugar consumption and find your own inner peace. But more than anything, it is about strengthening our bonds with friends and family, trusting in your own strength to successfully navigate this trial and embrace the idea that your future is now... your plans and dreams may now be placed front and center as your future "someday" is here today!"

—Mark Thomas

"Miss Wilms, THANK YOU for this beautifully written and deeply passionate read! This book is written from the heart in hopes of truly giving others strength and hope, regardless of where they are in their journey. I would also recommend that friends and family of cancer patients read this, so that you can better support those who are living this journey. This book is truly a gift!"

—Amazon Customer

"When reading this book I was frequently presented of a notion: here is a strong, independent, successful woman AND she is also a Cancer Survivor. I enjoyed the candid way she described the process of diagnosis and treatment including the real fears of losing hair, not being able to eat and treatment options. The part of the book that struck me the most was that the author learned to seek help, without pride or guilt. Although this journey was hard, the Author experienced it with an air of gratitude and honesty. She learned the advocacy and using her voice allows her to be part of the process not just the patient. It was a beautiful story about what connects us and separates but especially what makes us human. Her story of strength and perseverance is an inspiration to anyone who must go through this journey."

—Christi

"Anyone going through a breast cancer journey or who has a loved one going through it will benefit from Birgitte's frank account of her experience. Written with genuine warmth and openness, I found myself feeling as though she were right there placing a loving and supportive hand over mine while sharing her story and a cup tea. All of her sage advice and honesty regarding her options, and choices each step of the way is presented for the reader's empowerment and ability to self-advocate.

For those supporting a loved one with a diagnosis, they may find this beautifully written guide quite helpful in understanding what's happening and supportive for them as well.:"

—Sam Stanley

"Even though this book's title suggests an audience of those who have, or survived, breast cancer, I would highly recommend it for families and friends; it is an excellent insight into the struggles, mindset, and journey of a loved one who is stricken by this terrible disease. Additionally, Ms. Wilms' chapters on living life to the fullest and following your dreams are an inspiration to all, not just those who have had the misfortune of staring cancer in the face."

—Amazon Customer

"No one wants to diagnosed with breast cancer, but if it happens, nothing is more valuable than the helping hand of another survivor. As a 17-year survivor of high-grade breast cancer (and a fellow ocean enthusiast), I recognized much of Birgitte's story - and I so appreciated that this book told her WHOLE story - her warmth, her doubts and fears, her realism, and ultimately, her ability to be positive. This is not a book that will instruct you to be optimistic or brave all the time, and thank God for that. It's not overly filled with judge-y, lecture-y do's and don't's. It's also not a stale scientific text filled with unpronounceable words or latin names. Part autobiography, part advice book, this easy read will assure you that there is no wrong decision - and provide the quiet support needed to move through cancer so you can emerge on the other side knowing you've remained true to yourself."
—Allison Sallmon

"Ms. Wilms has created a literary marvel sharing her cancer journey and how she lived to tell the tale. It is both moving and inspirational, one you won't want to miss."
—Jennie Lynn
#1 Best selling author, *Magnetic Love*

"Even though this book's title suggests an audience of those who have or survived breast cancer, I would highly recommend it for families and friends; it is an excellent insight into the struggles, mindset, and journey of a loved one who is stricken by this terrible disease. Additionally, Ms. Wilms' chapters on living life to the fullest and following your dreams are an inspiration to *all*, not just those who have had the misfortune of staring cancer in the face."

—Jennifer Zunk

"As someone with personal experience with breast cancer, I can honestly say this book should be required reading for anyone diagnosed with breast cancer, anyone who knows someone with breast cancer or anyone who may get it. Birgitte has succeeded in communicating the complex emotions, pain, despair, fear and ultimately her triumph in a powerful and meaningful way. There are lessons to be learned for anyone reading her saga from dealing with the initial diagnosis to the complexity of treatment options and all the associated feelings and difficulties. However, where this story really shines in the profound sense of hope she communicates about living life after cancer. After reading this, you will be inspired to find renewed beauty in life and in living life nor just surviving."

What a heroic example of handling adversity – I will recommend it to everyone."

—Kathryn Codeiro

"Live Well beyond Breast Cancer is a candid journey through one woman's experience with diagnosis, treatment, and survival of breast cancer. Ms. Wilms writes with compassion, honesty, and transparency about her experience with a terrifying diagnosis. She encourages women to pay attention to their bodies and their inner voice. While medicine and technology make diagnosing cancer much more accurate sometimes cancer efficiently hides. Ms. Wilms discovered her own cancer by noticing and paying attention to changes in her body even though a mammogram indicated everything was normal. Upon diagnosis, Ms. Wilms leads the reader through her journey of feelings, fears, treatment options, medical teams, procedures, and recovery ever mindful that each cancer journey is unique and that every woman must make decisions that are right for her. Ms. Wilms also discusses the power of a gratitude practice, self-advocacy, healthful eating, and positivity. This is a book that is powerful to the woman who is facing this challenge, those that are in the process of treatment, those that are in recovery and those that support women who are, or have been, down this path. A difficult topic with a very hopeful message."

—Jenny Peterson, M.Ed.
Licensed Specialist in School Psychology

"Wow! I couldn't put this book down! *Living Well beyond Breast Cancer* is a reminder that with one diagnosis your life and those around you are forever changed. Ms. Wilms positive attitude is truly inspiring. For those going through canter treatment and those supporting loved one, this is a book for you. Use Ms. Wilms encouraging words and personal story to help you through. Great book! "

—Margie Laratta

To everyone who has contributed to the cause for a cure, especially the animals that involuntarily were put on this path to better humans' lives!

Contents

Chapter 1

And so It Begins

"Kites rise highest against the wind, not with it."
—Winston Churchill

This is my story to you as a cancer survivor who has just walked in the shoes you are about to walk in (or, you might already have those shoes on). My story is no more important than yours. It is not any more painful or scary or heroic, nor anything more or less than yours. It is simply my story, full of twists and turns. You will very likely recognize many similarities between my experiences and feelings and yours. No matter how the news of your diagnosis is presented, you are never quite prepared – and it is never good news. There is no way around it. But you have to find a way through, and I know you will. You absolutely will.

There are many steps to this journey. Communication with your medical team, your personal support teams, and other survivors will be some of your most valuable tools. My entire medical team was phenomenal, but nothing – absolutely *nothing* – could compare to or replace the value of a story, confirmation, or inspiration from somebody who has been there and who knows exactly how it feels. It could be the woman who is just a few steps ahead of you. She can shed invaluable light for you about the path you're both on. Even if your choices end up being completely different from hers, it doesn't matter. What matters is that she knows what you are about to or already going through. She has no ego or self-interest in your choice, only room for you to make your own choices with no judgment, even if it goes against her recommendations. It is a well-considered decision once you reach it, and she truly knows you made the decision that's perfect for you. All you had to do was consider her advice.

There were many extraordinary women along my way who I truly admired and whose contributions and stories I appreciated. One woman had been through many treatments, yet still showed up every time in full make-up or dressed up, along with her loving husband, for any seasonal occasion. They were a big testimony to living your life no matter how dire it may seem. One woman had a recurrence and experienced unthinkable complications that ended up being physically and emotionally costly – it was her story that I believe saved my life. Then there was a very young woman I talked to who was also going through cancer treatments. She had bandages over her medical port, so she had just been "hooked" up. She was bald and had no problems with it. She had a tank top on and happily showed off her healthy looking bosom. She told me she had just gotten a refill that day, and I could tell she was super pleased with how things were working out for her. I was so glad I got to speak with her and was so happy for her. I completely admired her and was inspired by her energy. She was that comfortable, much more so than I will ever be.

I was also lucky enough to have a friend of a friend to call when I was diagnosed. I had a lot of questions and was, of course, uneasy. She was a nurse and also a breast cancer survivor. I called her because I really trusted her in so many ways, and I was grateful that she was willing to speak to me. What I came to find out (and you will too) is that surviving women are more than happy to speak with women who have just been diagnosed. We know how helpful a survivor's voice is. We know you are nervous, we know it is daunting, we know you are scared, and we know what you are facing. We also know that you will get through this, even when the mountain ahead of you seems too big to climb.

When I needed help, the shiny brochures that presented the rotten news in a clinical manner weren't what I needed – it was the women's stories that outshined all of it. Those women had a phenomenal and powerful impact on me, more than I could have ever hoped. Because of them, I was able to make the absolute best choices for me – it was life-altering and life-saving all at the same time. Because of their winding roads that they happily shared with me, I have no hesitation to say they very much played a part in my life. They are why I will see my girls grow up to be women.

I'm sharing my story with you with the hope that, by telling you my story and reaching to you beyond the waiting room, it can hopefully have the same impact on your journey as the stories I heard had on mine. So, when you're reading, if some of the information doesn't apply to you, or it feels like too much, just skip it! It is good practice for you to learn how to put yourself first, if you aren't already. If I can send some light your way, inspire you, demystify and clarify this process, give you hope, help you believe and trust in yourself, help make you make decisions, make you laugh, make you relate, make you embrace, make you hopeful, or make your day – if there is any way I can touch your journey in a positive way – I will be tickled pink!

Chapter 2

So Much for Good Genes

*"Hope and fear cannot occupy the same space
at the same time. Invite one to stay."*
−Maya Angelou

I have been blessed with very good genes in many ways!
I am built like a typical Northern European – tall, fair,
blonde, and with little figure. My narrow hips very often
best fit men's clothes. Weight gain was never a problem,
but from time to time, I did have some extra pounds
I wanted to get rid of. When that happened, I would simply drink a sugar-loaded drink to trick my brain to think
I was full so I could skip a meal and get my stomach used
to being empty – a system override, sort of. This would
go on for about a week or so until I dropped the extra
weight I wanted to lose. I never counted calories or gave

up carbs. I lived a pretty healthy life overall, but I never joined a gym or health club.

Growing up in Denmark, exercise was something we really didn't schedule. We biked to school, walked to the train station, or simply went for a walk. After immigrating to the States, I spent close to three decades traveling the world and hosting underwater photography expeditions. It was a fabulous life and very active. Swimming around with an underwater camera is good exercise, especially when the impact was increased and the current was running. When possible, I would opt to swim back to the main boat rather than be picked up by the dinghy. After moving from Hawaii to Colorado, skiing was the winter activity, both downhill and cross-country, between dive trips. We did horseback riding and some jogging in the summer. Moving to New Hampshire, caring for our horses equaled a trip to the gym. The farm has a lovely trail system perfect for daily walks. Moving around a lot was just part of my day.

Plus, I was testing well on the medical side – mammograms, pap smears, you name it. I was acing it all. At forty years old, I decided to do a life screening to make a baseline for myself. Those results also came back favorable. My blood pressure was great, there was no clogging of the main artery, and my blood work came back great. The bad cholesterol was higher than they like it to be, but the ratio between the good cholesterol and the bad was in perfect harmony.

The nurse I saw said, "You have beautiful blood – you must eat like a horse." I kind of did. I have always eaten a ton and love to eat! I have never been a big fruit lover, but I did a lot of juicing and avoided high-cholesterol foods. On our underwater diving expeditions, we often visited the Solomon Islands and Papua New Guinea, both located in the South Pacific, and the villagers would bring their produce in their canoes to sell. We were blessed with freshly-picked papayas, bananas, and mangos when in-season between dives. We had it made. I gave myself a very strong and healthy base with home-cooked meals of chicken and fish, whole grains, etc., so I could enjoy some wine and desserts now and then. It was not a fancy or complicated diet – it was just good common sense. Everything was in moderation, and it worked great.

Though my mom was diagnosed with breast cancer and had a lumpectomy, I was not considered high-risk. As far as we knew, my mom was the only woman in our close family who was diagnosed. She was also diagnosed after menopause, so it was in a category where all women are simply at higher risk – it is just part of the deal of being a woman and alive. What I didn't know was that my biological aunt, who I never met, had died of breast cancer just three years before my diagnosis. This, of course, completely changed the picture. For some reason, she did not make it to the doctor's in time. I think she must have been scared and in denial. Apparently, it was too late when my niece realized how bad the situation was and tried to get her help. I can't help but wonder why, with all the modern medical treatments available, somebody would not go to the doctor. But sometimes, the truth might be more than we can take.

It was during one of the coldest winters on record in New Hampshire that I noticed a change. This is also when I was taking care of fifteen-plus horses and five dogs while being an owner of a 1791 house with all the charms that come with an antique home. I was logging some of the 260 acres we live on and had decided to have an additional five acres opened up in preparation for more retired horses coming to the farm. I was doing my real estate work and Airbnb-ing an apartment. I had also recently adopted an eight year old girl and taken in another foster child. The newest addition to our family was really tough, as she was far more traumatized than our first one. She didn't want to be in our family – she wanted to go back where she came from. It was really trying, and I was often in completely new parenting territory with no road map.

I was also going through menopause. Why wouldn't I be tired with everything I had going on? I was crazy to think otherwise. It was also no surprise that my work desk was really messy. I did not get around to cleaning it up because there were always a ton of interruptions – the phone, a dog that needed to come in. I rarely got five minutes of uninterrupted time. But there was one piece of paper that kept showing up from the local hospital. My annual mammogram was due. There had never been any issues in the past, so I decided I would call when I had the time, but after seeing the paper time and time again, I finally picked up the phone and scheduled an appointment.

During my daily routine, my showers were rushed. The water was really freezing in the dead of winter in central New Hampshire with negative temperatures for weeks on end; you wanted to get in and out as fast as possible, so I did not linger. One day, as I went about my business, I noticed that there was a change in my right breast. My nipple was going the wrong way. What the heck!? That was unusual. I felt no pain or discomfort though, and figured it was probably not that big of a deal. The tissue around it felt a little tense, but there were no lumps, so all was good. I had my mammogram scheduled anyway, so that would surely confirm I had nothing to worry about. I went back to being super busy, and honestly, wasn't all that concerned. But it nagged at me – my mom noticed an irregularity during a self-exam when she lifted her arms over her head. It was this self-exam that prompted her to make an appointment with her doctor, and that's when her cancer was found. That thought stuck with me

By the time the mammogram rolled around, things had changed a bit. My nipple was still strange and the area around it remained firm and was getting bigger. Maybe I was just more aware of it, but it was easily three inches across. I had myself convinced it was probably meno-pause-related "stuff." It was, after all, my first time going through menopause. Who didn't have surprising changes happen to their body, right? But it was very obvious that things were off at this time, and when I went into the examination room, I mentioned my observation to the nurse. She made a note for the doctor, but what really needed to happen was a diagnostic appointment which would be scheduled out a few weeks. I saw no reason for that. If they couldn't find anything wrong with my breast, as the area of concern was front, center, and blatantly obvious, an extra appointment would not really make any difference. Why push a possible diagnosis out any further?

So, I got the regular scans done with the usual discomfort. I went home and started dreading getting the letter in the mail with the results. But I was also so used to only good news, so I couldn't relate to what bad news would feel like. Because of that, I was able to not let the thoughts consume me, and after a week or so, the dreaded letter came in the mail – *negative!* No cancer found. I was not surprised – I was right and relieved! It was menopause "stuff," obviously, and my life went back to normal.

Then I started to notice that the area kept changing. My skin was getting red, and it was spreading just like an infection would. It reminded me of blood poisoning. There were now streaks of redness as well. Each week, the area changed and got bigger. I called my doctor and scheduled an appointment with her. We decided it was best to do an ultrasound. I was going on vacation soon, so I got a round of heavy antibiotics that would clear up this possible infection and prepare the area for correct and clear results from the ultrasound. My family and I went to North Carolina for winter break, where we walked the beaches and had a nice time. When it was time to go home, I was getting uneasy, as the redness had not changed. There had been no improvements.

I was relieved to go to the appointment at Dartmouth to find out what was going on. As I laid on the bed in my gown, things were starting to feel a bit different. There was a seriousness in the air, in spite of the sweetest nurse ever tending to me and a doctor who could not have been more pleasant. The room was dark, and the staff were fussing over me, making sure I had all the warm blankets I wanted and propping me up so I could be comfortable. There was no shortage of great care. I think they knew that my life was very likely about to change.

After my quick exam, my doctor did the ultrasound and left the room. He came back and said he was concerned. This was not what I was expecting. The mammogram had been clear, after all. He recommended a biopsy of the tissue and said I was welcome to reschedule if I wanted to digest the news... or we could do it now. Things were happening so quickly. I went for the biopsy right then and there and made a few calls. The room was getting pretty lonely. I had a great support system, but I was taking this step by myself. I was scared and confused, I hated needles, and I did not want to hear what I sensed was coming. The doctor was awesome and praised me for my decision – he even said I was brave. But I did not feel brave. I don't think anyone really does in the waiting period. It is an uneasy place, at best.

The results would be back in one or two days, and my doctor would call me personally. It sounded like he already knew, but didn't want to tell me before I had to drive home by myself. I made it home, talked it all over with Nancy, my life partner, and we just had to wait.

I was lucky because the waiting period for me was just one day before the call came in from my doctor. He was so sorry to inform me that it was, indeed, cancer – quite different news from the mammogram and not the news anyone wants to hear. I was by myself when I got the call, and it was one of those moments when it feels like life is staring you right in the face and there is no place to turn. The only option I had was to go straight through it. There are moments in this journey when you are by yourself and your life is very raw. This was one of those times! Every single woman, or anyone for that matter, who has received tough news knows this. It is a moment of truth, and it can feel very daunting, lonely, and overwhelming.

I don't how or why it happened, but gratitude started flowing and flooding over me. I was grateful for all the women who had gone through this before me. I was grateful for the doctors who had dedicated their lives to healing and curing. I was grateful that I was diagnosed now and not ten years earlier, as so much advancement has been achieved in just one decade. I was grateful for the donors and for all the people who have marched and contributed to the cure. I was grateful for my mom being an inspiration and staying strong and healthy. I was grateful for all the awareness around breast cancer. I was grateful for all the high-quality medical help that was available and within driving distance of me. I was grateful that I lived in the Western world, where my condition was detected, honored, and taken seriously. I was grateful I was listened to and respected by the members of my medical team I had met at that point. I was grateful I had taken matters into my own hands, paid attention to my body, and listened to the nagging voice I tried again and again to silence.

This state of gratitude turned out to be very healing and helpful, and it carried me very far in my journey. It might have been an unconscious choice. I might have grabbed the opportunity to hold onto gratitude before I grabbed onto fear or any other negative vibes. Once you take hold of an emotion, it becomes your walking stick, something we won't let go of even if it doesn't benefit us in any way, even if we know better. Gratitude was my self-defense mechanism, something positive to distract me, and, ultimately, something that would keep me on track before the fears would take over. It was very effective and very much one of the reasons I am here sharing my story with you.

I hope you will honor yourself and stay strong. Nobody knows you or your body as well as you do, and being your own advocate can be lifesaving. Lining up support from family and friends is great advocacy. Ask when you need help, even if you think you don't. Have another person with you to help you keep calm. This support is needed, so reach out. You will find that many are eager and willing to help. You might feel alone at this moment, but you are not. Please know I am right there with you. I know the punch in the stomach, the feeling of the blood draining into your feet, the complete disbelief. It can happen so quickly, and all these feelings are mixed in with each other. It is truly a whirlwind. If you feel overwhelmed, you are normal! I don't know of anybody who has not had their mind spinning going through something like this. This is a predictable and expected part of this chapter of your life. Some women question themselves, asking if they could have done more to prevent this and not be a burden to others. This is not a failure or a negative reflection of you. It might be the biggest stepping stone you ever get and a chance to propel yourself forward, so try and use it to your benefit.

Chapter 3

A Mountain of Information

"Attitude is a little thing that makes a big difference."
—Winston Churchill

So, I got the news – breast cancer. I was in a state of gratitude, but I did not embrace the situation as some women do. I already had a bunch of MRIs, CAT scans, and other tests done. Some were invasive with radioactive fluids injected into my veins. Plus, to have the most precise result, you can't move for about thirty minutes before the actual reading – and I had brought my knitting! How clueless was I! I had to go to the bathroom, but I could not find the door I had come out of. Then I saw a sign that read "Warning – radioactive!" Yep, that was me. That was my room.

My medical port, which I was told I was going to love, was installed on my left side. Usually, it is installed on

15

the right, but since my cancer was in my right breast, the port had to go on the left. It was an ugly bump under my skin, but I could appreciate that it would save my veins the trauma of being poked with needles each time I needed an infusion. It was very uncomfortable knowing that it was installed in one of the main veins going to my brain, and though I understood all the good reasons for its placement, I never fell in love with it.

After all the tests were behind me, it was time for me to meet my doctors. It was quite the schedule. The first appointment was with my surgeon. The door opened and the first thing I noticed was her hair – thick, brown, full, long, beautiful hair (really, Doc!?). It was really hard to like her and even harder not to like her. She was professional and extremely likable. She specialized in breast operations only, and because of her experience, she was able to give me the news. What I heard was, "Nobody dies of breast cancer anymore," (more on that later) but I had a long year ahead of me. Thinking back now, my situation was very serious, and when she learned I was leaning toward a mastectomy, she knew she didn't have to have "the talk" or try to convince me that a mastectomy was the minimum recommended treatment for my case. I was already there. I was also positive and so was she. Her nurse handed me a folder and when I skimmed the first sentences on each paper, it was obvious that attitude played a huge part in successful outcomes. It was refreshing that the doctor acknowledged they could try to cure, slice, and dice a body, but the spirit and outlook of the person was a very big part of the outcome.

Next, the door opened and the smiling nurse came into the room with her computer in her hand. Then, a thick ponytail of brown, shiny, healthy, thick curls that bounced up and down followed. Talk about putting salt into the wound! Just like my surgeon, she was really lovely which was almost irritating. It would have been easier not to like her. But she was fantastic, upbeat, and carried me through the appointment, and she prepared me to meet the oncologist. I was lucky to have her as my go-to person whenever I had any concerns or questions. I felt blessed.

Then, I met the oncologist, who was a very nice professional. We also had a common bond – horses. How we found out about this, I have no idea. Very likely, I wanted to change the subject and talk about something more pleasant than what I was facing. He tapped up and down my spine, looking for any hints of other solid masses should the cancer have spread. None were found, thank goodness. By this time, I was ready to put my clothes back on. Then, I had a timeline in hand. I don't really remember what the timeline was for even after it was written out. All I remember was the oncologist saying that the cancer could very likely have been hiding behind my nipple for years, maybe even a decade. The annual mammograms had done nothing to clarify the picture for me and early detection was wasted on me. The reality was that I had felt tired for a couple of years. I was napping more than

I should. It could easily be explained away that my days were too busy, but then again, who does not have busy days? It's clear to me now that my body was trying to keep the cancer at bay. I look at pictures from that time, and I can see the tiredness in my eyes.

My chemo would start right away. That shed some serious light on the situation. They were not waiting around. I remember a couple of my friends who had found lumps in their breasts and their doctors were not concerned. When I heard "cancer," I assumed there were quick action steps to handle the situation. It isn't necessarily so. There is so much that impacts this – the type of cancer, the advancement, the stage it is in. It became very clear to me that mine was really serious.

Next was the plastic surgeon. The receptionist was lovely and so were the nurses. A folder was handed to me, filled with flyers offering all kinds of options available to women diagnosed with breast cancer. I was able to take a peek at them. This was so hard to process and it put me in a new category. Prosthesis – really! Not an option. I could not keep track of my own keys, and for all I knew, it would end up under the bed and become a dog toy. Not for me. Then there were the implants. Another option I had no interest in. I knew of several women who got implants because they wanted a better look and experienced all kinds of troubles and complications. Not an option I wanted to entertain. I found a flyer explaining an option where breasts could be built from my own body tissue. I could live with that. Maybe that was not too bad after all. Finally, the door opened and the plastic surgeon came into the room. He was bald – finally! – and I could not have been happier. Or maybe he shaved his head – I couldn't tell and didn't care. Bald had never looked so good! We were trying to pinpoint where to go from here and what was best to do, weighing out all the pluses and minuses of each option. It was close to impossible to keep it all straight and hang on to all that was explained, but it was all explained to me very calmly and very patiently.

The nurses and the doctor all knew that my options were very limited, and they were trying to guide me so I could come to terms with the news little by little as the options kept decreasing. I was very upfront about the procedure I wanted. Why wouldn't anyone want to use their own tissue?

Measurements and pictures were taken, and the surgeon left the room. When he came back, I was given two options. Remove one breast and reduce the size of the other to make them match the best they could, or do a double mastectomy. Because of my healthy weight, there was not enough tissue for them to rebuild a breast with. It would be less than an A-cup, so this was not an option for me. Because the cancer was so close to the surface and in the skin, a skin graft could be necessary depending on how successful the treatments were. The skin to rebuild my new breast would be taken from my buttocks. What!? My butt as my boobs!? This was not going well.

I kept listening. If I didn't have enough tissue there, they would need to use some from my back. My nipples would be gone; they couldn't save them and rebuilding nipples had not been successful. However, a permanent tattoo was an option, though those would also fade over time and it would have to be redone approximately every five years. I would pick the new ones from a nipple portfolio.

This was all news to me and it was very overwhelming. A portfolio, to me, meant my photos. I realized in this whirlwind of information that I had very little say in next steps because of the advanced state of my cancer. I tried the best I could to come up with an idea of what I wanted, but quite frankly, I did not like any of the options, and this shined through in my responses. This was, by far, the toughest appointment of the day. My surgeon was very patient and made absolutely sure I understood what I had heard. I am sure I nodded my head, but to this day, I am not sure how much I actually heard. All I came up with was symmetry. Symmetry was important to me. That was my conclusion for this appointment. The rest I was still digesting and would continue to for months ahead. I did not have to come up with a decision that day – I had months to come to terms with it all – but it would take me that long to make a decision.

Because the cancer was right under the skin, I was a poster child for a clinical trial they were doing at Dartmouth. It was about the effectiveness of breathing a hundred percent oxygen in combination with radiation, and how it changed the effectiveness of the treatment. I could tell that they were anxious to have me sign up, though they tried not to put any pressure on me. But, I was a perfect candidate. How could I not say "yes?" I was following and benefitting from so many before me who had volunteered, so I happily agreed. They needed to insert a chip in the skin. At this point, I already had several metal beads in my breast from my first biopsy to mark where the tissue was taken from so they could keep track of each test. Now a chip too? I felt like my breast was turning into a junkyard! It was kind of funny, but in reality, it was hard to swallow. But my breast was going anyway, so what was the big deal? I might as well put it to good use. I was actually delighted to contribute to the cause. Because I got paid a small fee for participating, I then had to fill out financial forms along with all the consent and liability forms.

It was one of the nurses from one of my earlier appointments who also suggested I contact Joan. Joan was a breast cancer survivor herself, and she had a program called Cold Caps. These caps are known in Europe, and depending on what type of chemo you will receive, using them might give you a good chance to keep most of your hair. The caps would be between negative thirty-eight and negative forty-two degrees Fahrenheit. They would go on for an hour before the chemo started and three hours after. The idea was to restrict the blood flow to the hair follicles so they receive as little of the chemo as possible and result

21

in little hair loss. Frostbite could happened if we didn't cover up any bare skin. It must have been because of my long hair they mentioned it to me.

So, we called Joan since she lived close by the hospital. She was happy to see us and the Cold Caps were explained. This might seem crazy, but losing my hair was something I hadn't considered. Was I in denial? Was it just too much to process all at once? I don't know. So, I signed on with Jane right then and there, before I could even comprehend or think about the possibility of losing my hair. Jane had several sets of Cold Caps, and she funded all of them out of pocket. Not only that, it was very time consuming, and tons of coordination went into it, as she had a team of volunteers who prepared the huge coolers, blankets, etc. What a woman! What a team!

If you are interested, it would be worth your while to ask your medical team if they know about Cold Caps and if they are available. The nurses are far more knowledge about that than doctors, or at least that was my experience. Make sure your chemo treatments are given first, followed by any immunotherapy you might be receiving. The caps have to stay on for at least three hours after the last chemo, so it is the best use of time if those three hours are spent receiving other treatments rather than just waiting for hours to pass.

By the time we were done meeting everyone, I was utterly exhausted. Terms, new realities, and facts of life were swirling around. Timelines, options I didn't like, doctors I really trusted, medical trials, frostbite, nipple portfolios, skin grafts – and we hadn't even discussed radiation, which I knew also was coming. I was beat.

During my journey, I learned perspective, patience, and that a team of doctors, secretaries, nurses, technicians, and even cashiers can really make a difference, especially when you are super-sensitive and overwhelmed, frail and weakened by the side-effects, or just sick and tired of the whole ordeal. I can only hope you have a fantastic team of professionals like I had. I came to love all of them, and I am grateful beyond words for each and every one of them. I had no say, few choices, and no clue as to what was ahead of me. When I received my diagnosis, my path was laid out. My future doctors all knew when and where I would be for the next twelve months. My diagnosis was that clear: stage 3 breast cancer, and it was on the move. It was very serious, but, ironically, it was that exact movement that ended up saving my life. The professionals all treated each appointment with patience and tip-toed the delivery of the news as gently as they could.

My team was beyond wonderful. When my diagnosis was detected, my treatment plan was scheduled out. I had a clear sense of the coordination between the doctors. It was both very specific to me and also very specific to the diagnosis. Many teams from all the different departments went out of their way to coordinate when at all possible to make my trips fewer and my days shorter. They helped in any way they could to make the outcome the very best it could be. There is no way around it: stage 4 breast cancer is serious business, and their personal touch and extra efforts were mind-boggling and extraordinary. It was like a well-oiled machine, which I deeply appreciated. You need to be in good hands when handling treatment, and I felt that very strongly.

There was an unexpected blessing in the most unlikely place of all: the oncology waiting room at Dartmouth (K3, to be exact). This was where I spent many hours waiting for my turn for treatment. It is not a very uplifting place at first glance, a waiting room of tired and balding people. At the same time, it is also where family stepped up to the plate, where inspiring stories were heard, and where people happily showed up with appreciation for their treatments, because those infusions were the reasons they were still here and the reason they were still fighting. It is a mixed bag of high emotions, to say the least. But the waiting room, for me, was where I met three women who shaped my path and helped me make what I believe to be a life-saving decision when I needed help the most. This incredible guidance was beyond the brochures, statistics, and all the confusing professional lingo.

A little bit of reading ahead of time might prepare you for some of the terms, realities, and onslaughts of information that might be coming your way. I gathered from other cancer patients they had similar experiences. One woman described determining her treatment plan as being put in front of a firing squad, and there really is some truth to that. So, know this might also happen to you. I don't really believe you can prepare for it all, but so many terms and ideas will be presented to you all at once, I recommend that you stick with the information your doctor's office gives to you. If you can get their information prior to the appointment, that would be helpful.

I don't know if doctors will provide this information ahead of time. I can imagine it would differ from doctor to doctor. Some "light" informational material that at least gets your mind in the right direction ahead of time can make all the information more comprehensible. For me, it was too much at one time and I simply could not digest it all at once. Try and avoid this happening to you. I truly hope you will have a friend or loved one – somebody who can advocate for you and, most importantly, be there for you and listen to all that is being said and explained. Taking notes is a really good idea. Hopefully, this book has already introduced you to some terms you are not familiar with and is helping to prepare you. This is a very big day. The bad news is that it's one of hardest and the good news is that it is now over with! You will have lots to "digest," but you are through one of the biggest hurdles already.

Chapter 4

Crash Course

"It is just a bad day, not a bad life."
−Unknown

After my diagnosis, I realized I had far more to learn than I ever knew or anticipated. You might find this to be true for you too. One of the many eye-opening revelations I had is that the operation often comes first. It is the "most desirable" option, as it is a good sign that the cancer is small and easy to operate on. If it is not, chemo will likely be the first step as an attempt to get the cancer contained, shrunk, or maybe even gone altogether. Some women have radiation, some receive chemo "only," and some have both. Some women have an operation, chemo, and radiation – the lovely trio! I was that person. My mom was as well, so I was under the assumption that this was the normal course for all breast cancer patients.

This is not true, not even close. The more women I met, the more I realized how different each of our paths were. Some were operated on and were given radiation "only." Some had chemo and no radiation. The variety of options was surprising to me, and I was so happy for them because their side effects were far less. That is often more the case than not. I only met one woman who underwent all the operations and treatments I did. It was also in the waiting room, and she was an unbelievable trooper. I wish we had kept in touch. I would love to know she got through. She really needed a friend, and quite frankly, I did too at that point.

It is extremely important to have a clear understanding of what is going on and why appointments are scheduled in the order they are. This journey will very likely be a crash course for you, as it is for most of us. I thought I had learned a lot from my mom's complicated journey. Hers ended up a horrible mess due to the side effects that kept turning into other issues unrelated to the cancer, but I did come into this journey with some hands-on experience and some real ideas on what would happen because of that. However, Mom was in Denmark. She had a lumpectomy ten years before I was diagnosed, so my path was still very different that hers.

It's really important to find out about the margins of the lump. If the lump is "just" a lump, it can be there for years without making a move. This was also a surprise to me, but it made sense and it also explained why some of my friends who had a lump or found a suspicious area had contacted their doctor. Even after it had been confirmed it was cancer, the mood and pace were very casual as they moved forward.

I know mammograms save lives. There is no doubt about it, and I don't recommend that mammograms should not be done. But I can't help but wonder how many lives the mammograms actually claim by giving a false reading of "negative" and false sense of security when cancer is actually alive and well. I am convinced that women have gone untreated who should have been seeing a doctor immediately, instead of waiting another year for their next preventative mammogram. According to my oncologist, the tissue behind the nipple is very dense, and my cancer could easily have been hidden there and missed for years, perhaps even a decade. That makes sense, but what about the three-inch area around it? It was, after all, obvious to the eye that point – how could this area not show up? This area lit up like a Christmas tree on the MRI and showed up very clearly on the ultrasound. An MRI is very expensive and my insurance only covered part of the cost. It is also a bit invasive, as it is, after all, radioactive material that is injected into your vein. It would, however, be wonderful if one day, everyone could be examined with an ultrasound. I can only guess that it is cost that prevents us from having this as an option for our preventable care. The good news is that self-exams are very effective and free! I know tons of women now that discovered their cancer during a self-exam. My mom detected her own irregularity when she lifted her arms over her head. It was because of this I unwillingly paid attention to my irregularity.

Breast cancer shows up in so many ways. It can actually show up in the stomach – I didn't know that! I thought it was more a one-size fits all treatment, and when cancer was detected, the trio applied for all breast cancer patients. It is important to know that the trio might not apply to you – and this is good news. From what I could tell, most of the survivors I have met have had far less treatments than me. It is still a lot to take in, regardless of your diagnosis, type of cancer, and what stage it is, but the lesser advanced diagnosis, the lesser possible side effects and length of treatments. There has been so much advancement in this field, and they have gotten so good at pinpointing the different cancers. Along with early detection, it has almost become routine. Focusing on all the great stories and successes there are will help keep your mind positive. The black cloud is a lot lighter now than it used to be for women diagnosed.

You know your body best, and you know how you feel at your best. Even you are unsure or notice a difference or a change in how you feel, don't brush if off as menopause, or "I am sure I am fine – I'll get to it later." As women, we are way too quick to put everyone else's priorities ahead of ours. I know I was tired, and I was getting more and more tired all the time. It was noticeable, but I explained it away, and, combined with a mammogram that confirmed it, I believed all was well. It almost claimed my life. I was lucky that it was under my skin and I could see it just by looking at it. I could see it changed, that it was moving, and that something wasn't right. If I hadn't noticed, I am not sure what shape I would be in today. I am so glad I had the courage to question what my body was going through and that I didn't move forward in blind faith, believing that the professional conclusions were more valid or correct than my own observations. I'm glad I questioned it. I saved my own life, and now my girls still have me. Pay attention for you and your loved ones, and put yourself first.

Chapter 5

Eat Your Vegetables

"You are what you eat."
–Anthelme Brillat-Savarin

For all we know, many of us already have cancer cells in our bodies. If we have healthy lifestyles and get the sleep we need to heal, we fight the cancer successfully every day. There is no doubt that our lifestyle choices contribute to our bodies' ability to successfully conquer the free radicals. Cancer is no longer an old person's disease. It is a known fact that younger and younger women are getting diagnosed with breast cancer. It is vital that we are active in detecting it, because being young is no longer a good reason to believe you are not at risk. Information varies depending on where you find it, but around 250,000 women are being diagnosed on an annual basis. Childhood cancer is also on the rise. It simply has to do with our unhealthy lifestyle. We still do not put enough emphasis on prevention.

Dr. Laleh specializes in dietary prevention of cancer, and I was lucky enough to participate in her course as part of the twelve-week rehabilitation "Bridge Program" I attended. I was only able to attend half of the program, but I was still aghast at what I learned and what our foods really consist of. Dr. Laleh put this program together because she lost her father to stomach cancer. Her life was completely impacted by the loss, and though she had not had cancer herself (a testimony to her program) she was still as compassionate as if she herself was a survivor. "We don't have a health care system; we have a sick care system," she said. She is so right.

I was raised in Denmark and was shocked when I first came here and saw Americans' habits around food. Dr. Laleh was born in Iran and one of the first shocks she had as a foreigner was the American breakfast. It is more like dessert than a healthy meal to kick off the day with. She went into depth about sugars, GMOs, food coloring, and because of that information, I have changed a lot of my habits to a much healthier diet.

The American lifestyle (and European, to a lesser extent) have surrendered to the fast food tradition, not just with drive-thrus, but by eating meals in the car and "stick-it-in" microwave meals. Sugary cereals with eye-catchingly bright colors are lined up on the shelves for our kids to choose from. But the colors cause cancer and all the sugars feed the cancer cells. Talk about cancer in a box! This is considered good food, and I know some of these cereals are even served at my girls' school. There is a surprising food insecurity throughout the United States, and a meal, cancer-causing or not, is considered better than no food at all. So, they figure, at least the kids get a meal and won't go hungry.

And what about all the sugars and colorings in soft drinks (which I refer to as liquid candy)? Or the colors in highly processed chips or neon-orange cheese puffs? It is poison and creates a good environment for cancer to start and then flourish. No wonder cancer is on the rise in all generations. Consider the quality of the meat we eat as well. Stressed-out animals create stress hormones in themselves – how unhealthy is that for our bodies? We have also altered the genetics of animals so they grow, in some cases with deformities, so the producers can meet a specific demand. The chicken is a good example. Some of them have chests so big, the poor animal can't reach the ground of the cage.

Then there are GMO foods – these are pretty much impossible to get around. The all-American delicious sweet corn is full of GMOs. If you don't want to eat it, then say goodbye to corn on the cob at the summer BBQs, tortillas, and tortilla chips. The FDA recently recommended that a warning should be put on the labels that cheese is carcinogenic. Yes, cheese! All this and more

I learned from Dr. Laleh's program, and it truly is just scratching the surface.

What really shocked me is when Dr. Laleh started talking about dairy's impact on our health and the many misconceptions we have about our diet. In Denmark, we didn't have the fast food tradition, but we did drink milk (and a lot of it) to get strong bones. No water – water was for the plants. Growth hormones are also naturally found in milk. It is for the calf so it can survive and grow quickly. It is nature's way to prepare prey animals for survival, so they can outrun a predator. But there might also be added antibiotics and additional growth hormones in the meat. I just can't help but wonder if the milk contributed to cancer flourishing in my body.

So, what can you do? Have water instead of a soda. Start liking green tea, which has great antioxidants. I can't stand the taste personally, so I mix it in with my other teas to trick myself. There are all kinds of small things that can be done. White processed sugar has no place in your diet. It is one of the worst foods. Stevia, is a natural herb, and a great sweetener with zero calories. Go to the local farmer's market and buy your honey and meat there. It is usually a bit pricier, but you don't need as much as you think. Make sure to rest and then rest some more.

Eat your vegetables – truthfully. The greens are super-foods and they are recommended regardless of any diet. They are loaded with calcium, in case you're wondering where the calcium will come from if you decide to give up dairy products. Many cultures don't have dairy in their diet. Japan and countries in the South Pacific are good examples of this – they eat a lot of greens. As a matter of fact, the villagers hustle around when the *dimdims* (which means strangers) visit their villages, in case a coconut falls from a tree. Our skulls would break from the impact, yet they are not concerned about their own skulls breaking. Interesting, isn't it? And they don't have a drop of milk in their diet. There are so many simple steps that can be done, but few are actually acting on them.

Another part of my lifestyle I had to change after my diagnosis was getting more rest. I no longer compromise here. Nowadays, there always seems to be a notification or post to follow. Society is always on the go. The younger generation especially never gets a chance to turn off the world. It is very fast-paced, but it has been proven again and again that proper rest and time-off is helpful to the human body and spirit. It creates happier people and increases productivity. Rest is absolutely vital to the body's self-healing, but many do not go a night without interruption because they have their phone with them in bed. It is vital to our health to take breaks from this every single day and make time for some "me" time. Put it on your calendar, and make sure to obey the "me time" appointment every day for at least thirty minutes.

There is so much you can do to stay healthy and active. It can be as simple as going for a walk, run, hike, or to the gym. Cancer can't grow well in an oxygen-rich environment, so taking time for you is so healthy. A long walk in the woods can clear your mind and inspire you. Be by the water – it cleanses. For me, nature is essential. I have to be in it to thrive. If you do not have access to nature right outside your door, plant a garden or get some potted plants. Treat yourself to fresh-cut flowers and enjoy a beautiful flower arrangement. Get a bird feeder and enjoy the birds coming to your home. Sit in the sun, breathe fresh air. This will all lift your spirit.

You should also consider planning something to look forward to after all the treatments as part of your self care. Once all is said-and-done, you should celebrate this occasion and yourself. It will distract you from your current situation, give you a very specific event to focus on, distract your mind, and put your attention on the future. It can be planning a weekend on the beach, taking time to paint for an entire week, or going on a retreat. For me, it was the Andrea Bocelli concert in Boston with an overnight stay. The logistics were very manageable. I could not wait, and I spent hours looking forward to it. It was a great choice for me – his voice was overwhelmingly powerful, and it was absolutely a fantastic and healing night. So, I recommend whatever you choose be nurturing and relaxing. Running a marathon or summit a mountain peak are not good goals at this time.

Living healthily is considered time-consuming and costly for a lot of people, and compared to the lifestyle many are living, they are right. They don't know any differently or how to change. Once, a farmer friend of mine gave some of his fresh vegetables as a donation to our local food pantry and they rotted away because nobody knew how to cook them. That is how far off-track we have gotten.

But cost is not just a dollar amount. Think of the meals you don't cook together with your family – it's a huge missed opportunity to bond and create a rhythm in your life. Think of all the time you could have spent cooking, and it is now spent in the car going back and forth to the hospital! Think of the cost of the treatments and the emotional toll on you and your loved ones. Make the necessary changes, and the sooner, the better. Do it for your loved ones, the animals, and the planet – and absolutely do it for you too! Taking care of yourself is an investment in you and in your future. You are worth the time and the effort! Treat yourself to something special, and treat yourself kindly.

Chapter 6

The Big Hairy Facts and Other Issues

"Do not let what you cannot do interfere with what you can do."
—John Wooden

When talking about cancer and chemo, the topic of hair and other strong side effects comes up. It can't be avoided, as much as we would like it to be. Hair is a particularly interesting topic. The more you dig into the subject, the more interesting it gets.

Regardless of the country or culture, hair plays a huge role in a human's beauty, identity, and power. We have about five million hair follicles, and 100,000 of those are on our heads. That's an impressive number, and it is also one of the traits that makes us mammals – it makes us who we are. There is a surprising amount of identity wrapped into your hair. It might surprise you how much – I know it surprised me, even after going through this process with my mom.

I am naturally blonde and was born with thin hair. It was quite the curse. I grew up with the belief that if you cut your hair short, it will get thicker. So, I was encouraged to keep cutting it so I could get thicker hair. My mom used to bring a wet sponge with her for when the baby portraits were taken, so I wouldn't appear bald (the family pride was at stake here). She continued to bring the sponge with her way beyond infanthood. I ended up embracing my thin hair and it turned out to be quite practical for me.

My hair would dry quickly in-between dives. When you dive three to seven times a day, being dry for just a split second is really nice. My pony tail was like built-in A/C – keeping it wet when going to the hot airport in the tropics was a blessing. I was recognized in the water from long distances away. My floating golden locks were worrisome on shark feeds, as it could easily be mistaken for some floating white fish chuck (but I was never a fan of these shark feeds anyway). When I was diagnosed with breast cancer, it never dawned on me that I would lose my hair. Maybe I was in a state of denial, or perhaps I was so surprised by the news – and things moved so quickly – I never could truly take the time to wrap my head around the consequences. I was already very aware of the whole process, as I had lived through it all with my mom. Maybe knowing how well she handled it and how great she looked bald gave me peace. I am not sure.

When Joan, the founder of the Cold Cap program in our area, got her diagnosis, she said she was terrified. She had two questions: "Am I going to die?" and "Am I going to lose my hair?" Both questions were terrifying. We all know that the hair will grow back at some point, but it can still feel unimaginable to think of yourself as bald. The outside world may or may not get used to seeing you bald, but seeing yourself in the mirror is a moment of truth. Some women proudly show their shaved head in public. I envy them. I will never be one of them. Gratitude and all, I was not that big. In some cases, family members shave their heads in support of a loved one. How wonderful it must be to have such a level of loving support! I am not sure if I could do that. Maybe if one of my girls got breast cancer, it would be a consideration, but even then, I am not so sure.

Joan's fear of losing her hair was her reason for starting the Cold Cap program. It costs thousands of dollars for a set of six caps. They are put on dry ice to reach the most effective desired temperatures (somewhere between negative thirty-nine and negative forty-two degrees Fahrenheit). Some women can't tolerate the cold temperature. Even I have to admit, after hours and hours of wearing them, it got cold – and old. The first one was the hardest, and then I got the pre-meds, which contained a big dose of Benadryl. Needless to say, I was half asleep for most of the time it was on. It was really Nancy that was putting in the effort. The caps were changed every twenty minutes, and when it was done, they were put back into the cooler with the dry ice to be cooled down until the next round. I was nicely tucked in under the electric heated blanket so I was all set for the first part of the day.

It is really important that the chemo is given first. The caps have to be worn three hours after the chemo treatment, so you don't want the chemo to be the last treatment and then add another three hours to the day. Pre-meds, chemo, and then immunotherapy with wait times in between is ideal (we were always the last patients to leave the hospital anyway). Usually, my infusion days would start at 8 a.m. or so, and we would leave around 7 p.m. The days were long for sure.

The Cold Caps were effective, but not as effective for me as they were for others. Had I been inside the three week timeframe prior to starting the first chemo (where I could have cut my hair), I might have had more success. The hair follicles experience trauma when we cut our hair, and it can compromise the hold the follicles have. My chemo was happening within two weeks, so I missed this deadline. I experienced some shedding, which was expected. I did also lose a band of hair around where you keep your sunglasses when you want them out of your face. But I told myself that the long bangs I used to cover this bald area with was just right. After the fifth chemo treatment, I was bed-ridden and most of the hair I had left rubbed off. It was still worth the effort, and though my hair was super thin, I had enough hair to tell myself I was doing great!

While this was happening, we also had a big issue brewing. We'd taken in a beautiful little foster child, but this beautiful girl could be taken away from us. She was not ours yet. There is always an element of uncertainty until the adoption is final. I was not sure where the state would stand if they knew of my diagnosis. So I decided to pretend all was well.

It was going to be really difficult to keep it quiet, but I would do all I could so this little beautiful girl would not be passed off to yet another temporary home. If the Cold Caps didn't work, I would be bald when entering the courtroom on the adoption day. It would be very hard to pretend all was well if I showed up bald. When the court date rolled around, the Cold Caps were somewhat effective, but the hair loss was getting obvious. I think it was less than a week after the second infusion, so I could pull it off – but it would be extremely close. Finally, the judge said the adoption was irreversible, and no sweeter words have ever been spoken. The hammer slammed, and it was a done deal. We went out for ice cream, and then I went back home and right to bed. It had been an awesome day. I was a mom for the second time.

Hair loss is one of the biggest side effects of chemo, but there are other side effects that need to be dealt with as well, and it is hard to know how to prepare for the unknown. It felt like my body was saying "What did I do wrong?" after I got my first chemo treatments. I kept a diary so I could get a baseline of my new normal. After five days, I would start to get sick to my stomach. The accumulative effects of the treatment were very real, and with each round, the side effects worsened. The period of times when I was sick to my stomach got longer each time. After the fifth treatment, I had lost eighteen pounds, mainly due to diarrhea, which was a lot to lose for me. The prescription medication they gave me for nausea and diarrhea didn't work at all. I couldn't even smell food without my stomach starting to act up. It would kick my stomach in overdrive and I would fly out of the room. It took me awhile to be able to handle anything cooking in the oven. It was too much food smell to deal with and overwhelmed my senses.

Everything tasted salty. Even coffee tasted like it was made with salt water. So to override the salty taste, I chose salty food.. Fruit surprisingly tasted better. It was delicious! My stomach couldn't handle a lot, but at least fruit was something I could look forward to.

It is a good idea to economize what you consume. I recommend you don't eat your favorite foods while going through the chemo treatments. Enjoy your favorite dishes after you are all done, or you most likely won't like them during or after. That's what happened to me. I struggled for months after treatment with some of my very favorite dishes. The taste, smells, and textures all bothered me. Rice felt like a sticky mess and ground cooked beef reminded me of eating hairy ticks (for lack of better words). I had no idea this would happen, and it took me a long time afterward to like rice again (and even longer to like tacos).

If you are reading this book before starting chemo, that is great. Please be sure to have lots of different foods on hand. They should be soft and easy on your mouth, like almond yogurt, baked potatoes, avocados, hummus, miso soup (if you are HERS negative), bananas, etc. What you can eat one moment can make you sick the next and this change happens very quickly. So, have all the foods you can handle available at all times, so you can grab them right when you need them. When you feel like eating, you should be eating. Nurture your body as much and as often as you can handle.

All my side effects were as predicted. They were pretty severe, but not out of the ordinary. I was lucky because my mouth didn't turn into a blistering mess. I was worried it would after the first round, and I am grateful it never happened. But my mouth did get very sensitive – even my teeth and lips were sensitive. The wrong toothpaste and lip balm would send me through the roof. It had to be mild with no peppermint. As time went on, I tried to supplement my diet with protein drinks and found a great plant-based brand.

After drinking this, it came back up on two different occasions – once at home and once on the bathroom wall while I was out showing a house. I should never have been out, but I was holding onto the fact that some patients can work and keep their normal schedule during the treatments. On my way home, I had to pull over several times, and luckily, it was all on quiet country roads. Pulling over was easy. I couldn't stomach that brand of protein powders any longer, so I went to a store brand, but then when I took one sip of the "off the shelves" protein drink, my mouth was on fire. The overwhelming amount of sugar just burned my tongue and gums, and I never took another sip. It was downright painful! Yogurt, which is considered a healthy meal, but was just as filled with sugar, had the same burning effect in my mouth. It was shocking. Again, sugar is one of the absolute worst foods anyone can eat – and it is everywhere! Please avoid these foods. They do not serve you! Avoid lip balm and tooth paste with peppermint and other strong oils. They can easily burn your already sensitive mouth.

I was advised to drink sixty-four ounces of water after each treatment to lessen the side effects. As soon as the chemo was injected, it was doing its job, and then when it was done, it was time for me to get rid of it. The sooner that stuff got flushed out of my body, the better. The body will do its best to quickly break the chemicals down so the chemo will no longer be chemo, and the more you drink, the better off you are. Ask your oncologist or one of your nurses what your recommended amount of water is. It really helps ease the side effects. For me, it was nice to know I could actively participate in my own recovery. There were steps I could take to make life easier. I suggest you get a water bottle with ounces marked on the side. Have as many as you need in the right size on hand prior to going to the hospital.

Be easy on yourself. I, no doubt, pushed myself far past my capability and what was best for me. I kept hanging on to what I had read in one of the materials I was given. I happily noted that some patients can work full-time and keep their normal schedule throughout the treatments. I thought that was great and tried to do it too. Then when my health really buckled, I questioned myself. Why was I such a "baby?" I was the healthy one, and though I had expected side effects, why could some keep on going at a normal pace? It was very confusing. I finally asked one of the nurses. She looked at the two chemo drugs I was receiving, and said, "You are being treated with not one but two very strong chemo drugs. They are hitting you really hard." That explained it. After the third and fourth rounds of chemo, my skin would get a nasty rash and I noticed my eyesight was getting worse. These treatments *were* hard. I could finally ease up on myself. I had to stop trying to do as much as I did. It was not helpful to me or my family, seeing me that compromised yet still up and about.

There are times when you want to contribute and feel "normal," but it is really more important to get through this period. It is temporary. This is hard to remember,

I know, but it is also a fact. So, take your naps if you have to. Don't push beyond your new limits – there is no need to. Instead, listen to your favorite music. Find the best blanket to snuggle under. Give yourself permission to do whatever is necessary to completely heal. You will be better off in the long run. There is no need to make this harder than it has to be.

I wish I had had a better understanding of the side effects specific to my treatments. I came into this journey thinking the worst. After reading the materials, I was so happy to find out this was not so, which was great and also surprising. I was planning on horseback riding, doing my daily morning walks, feeding the horses, being a mom – just to find out that my treatments were on the top list for severe side effects. I gave myself a hard time when I buckled, without realizing this was normal. Chemo treatments are not all created equal. So, please, be sure to ask what to expect. Each patient is different, and we will all react differently. But there are facts about each chemo drug that you should know about going into it. It is vital to your planning ahead, not just for you, but also your support system. It is so helpful to have realistic expectations and the chance to prepare yourself mentally. You are entitled to know about your treatments. So ask, ask, and ask. The one silver lining is that if you receive a harsh chemo and you get sick as a dog – it is very likely super effective and doing its job!

Chapter 7

So Done!

*"Don't worry about the darkness, for that
is when the stars shine the brightest."*
—Napoleon Hill

Gratitude really helped keep me afloat emotionally. It was also a great state of mind to be in. I had so much to be thankful for. I had Nancy's support, and my brother came to visit twice! That had never happened before. My parents came to help out and stayed for months, which was beyond wonderful. I had my dogs, and there was the wonderful fact that I pulled off the adoption. I had a lovely extended family that kept checking in on me and friends nearby that also offered great support. In the early stages of chemo, I would walk on my trails. I even jumped on my horse when I no longer could do my daily walks. I could enjoy the view of my pasture swinging from my hammock. All things considered, I was indeed blessed, and I gave thanks every day.

But it was when I stood up while on the "throne" and gave thanks that I managed to get up and on my knees in time to vomit that I decided I was taking the gratitude too far. It was turning into madness, and I was not listening to myself. It was becoming hard to stay close to my intuition and my gut feelings. It felt like chemo put a grey fog in between my body and my soul, and I only had access to my soul every once in a while when the fog eased up. But at that moment, I was connected and it was clear – I was *done trying to be grateful!* I had no more energy to keep up my good spirit. I had no more to give. And if I had the sixth and last chemo, it would land me in the hospital. I knew my body couldn't take anymore. What was the point of being so weak right before my big operation? It is serious business to not finish all the treatments. I was not willing to take any risks, mainly for my family's sake, and though I had made my decision, it was not cast in stone until I spoke with my surgeon and my oncologist.

The day was a defining moment for me. As we got to the main entrance, I realized I could no longer walk to my doctor's office. It was very hard to have a "stand tall" and "chin high" attitude when my body could no longer keep me upright. As I reached for the wheelchair, I finally surrendered to being sick. It took me a very long time to get to this point, and I did not give it up easily. Quite frankly,

I would have been kinder to myself if I had surrendered sooner. I should have allowed myself to ask for help

I was rolled into my surgeon's office, and she was awesome as usual. I told her of my decision, but I wanted to talk to her first before the decision was final. I would do the last chemo if I had to, but it seemed to me that I would be at high risk going into surgery by being completely weak. I knew that I would have a month of rest between the last chemo and the operation, but I was not willing to take any chances or risks for my daughters' sake. They had already experienced so much loss, and quite frankly, as miserable I was, I was not done living either.

When I asked my surgeon if the operation would be any different if I didn't finish the scheduled chemo, her answer was no. It would be the exact same operation regardless. She could not give me the thumbs up, however – that was up to my oncologist. As luck would have it, my next appointment that day was with him. So, the nurse showed up with her lovely curly ponytail and big smile, as usual. I talked to her about my decision, and she assured me I absolutely had to do the last chemo. There was no way around it, but she would check with the oncologist. It was not looking good for me, and I dreaded the next few weeks already. It is daunting to know the medication that will cure you will also bring you right to the breaking point. When she came back in, she made a cross with her hands in front of her chest. I had gotten the doctor's blessings. And just like that – I was done with chemo! The side effects would linger, but I was moving forward and was on my way to put them all behind me. The operation would be in a month! My head was spinning, and it was such great news – I felt light for the first time in a long time. The biggest chapter was behind me. I had a month off from any treatments – I was on cancer treatment vacation and it was time to recharge as much as possible and get a break. I felt the worst was truly over.

The best part was that my parents and brother had come over to stay for a couple of months right at that time as well, so I could enjoy their company. I felt bad because they came due to my severe side effects, and now I was on the other side of it. I felt like I had misled them, but as it turned out, their help was absolutely needed. It was really nice to have them staying for this length of time for the first time since I left Denmark three decades earlier. It was a wonderful treat, and the timing ended up being great after all.

The rest was nice and needed, and I probably went to some appointments that I can't remember. What I do remember is the night before my surgery. It snowed and snowed and snowed. My house is a forty-five minute drive on winding and hilly back roads, and we literally slid our way to the hospital. I was sure we were late, but once again, the hospital knew what they were doing. When we got there, there was a long line. That was the first time I saw that, and I was in a panic, but we got through and had plenty of time prior to being called in. I can reflect now on how lucky I was to have both my mom and Nancy there with me. I was so grateful for the support. I felt blessed.

When I was called in, I met the anesthesiologists. Forms were signed, and I was once again impressed with the time they took to explain everything. I can just imagine how many times they have to go through this, and yet I never felt rushed or any impatience from their side. Everything was done in the most professional manner. Looking back, what I wish I had asked for beforehand was to be completely out cold when I entered the operation room. When they wheeled me in, I got a glimpse of all the operation tools, and it was one of the worst moments for me. It was very unnerving.

Please keep that in mind for yourself. I don't know how you feel about surgical tools or needles, but the added stress of seeing them was not great. From then on, I don't remember anything, and I am glad. If you are as adverse to the operation room as I am, I recommend and hope you will bring this to the anesthesiologist's attention. I found they were more than willing to help out, and they were dedicated to easing the stress of the situation. They welcomed the opportunity to do whatever they could to make it the best possible experience for me.

Nancy and my mom were kept abreast on how the operation was proceeding. My surgeon would remove one breast and move to the second one while my plastic surgeon would start inserting the temporary expanders (more on that later). It was a team effort, and I really appreciated that these two operations could be done simultaneously. Everything was going well. Nancy later relayed to me that my surgeon had come out after it was all done and I was out of the operation room, and she was sincerely happy with the outcome. She was elated actually, as happy as if it had been her own sister. There is no way to describe the wonderful feeling when a professional, who has your life in their hands, is sincerely invested and interested in your outcome and in your well-being.

I was very sorry I missed that moment, but I was lucky enough that she came to me the next morning to check in and congratulate me. The other great news was that my reaction to the chemo had been phenomenal! It was so successful that no skin graft was necessary. Now that was huge and good, obviously! There was no cancer in the four lymph nodes, which they were concerned about. A more detailed test would be done other than the one done during the operation, but since that initial test came back negative, they were very optimistic that would also be the case for the more detailed and precise test. And they were right – I was cancer free!

My friend and cancer survivor Janet had a heck of a time losing her one breast. As a matter of fact, she couldn't bear to look at herself for over a week. After my surgery, I looked down my shirt right away, and I already had some bumps that looked just fine. I was well on my way. What I didn't know was that the temporary expander would be very uncomfortable, and I was in a lot of pain the first few days. I also had the fluid drains on each side, and I was told the more I moved my arms, the more drainage, which meant the longer I had to have them in. I did everything in my power not to move my arms – they were pretty much glued to my sides, and the drains were removed exactly a week afterwards, which was quick

Then came the compression bra. It was very restrictive, but it didn't last that long either. I was far from the bra size I was prior to the mastectomy, and it was a goal to get close to my natural size. So, I showed up for my first refill. I am not very good with needles, so I took one look at the needles with the tubes attached in the tray and hoped they had been left there from the previous appointment and were not meant for me. I was, of course, wrong, and the needles were inserted in my chest – I was going to have fifty CCs put into my chest. The refills are done in certain amounts of CCs so the muscles and other tissues can handle the expansion. My boobs are measured in CCs now and not bra size.

Once the appointment was over, I knew I was not coming back for any more refills. I made that very clear. I didn't care how big I was. I was absolutely done, beyond a shadow of a doubt. My size was not at all important. I was symmetrical and I had boobs – mission accomplished. I pulled the plug on all future refills. I'd had it with the expander in my body – it was like wearing a plastic bra with underwires that were too small. There was no way to get comfortable. But I knew the plastic surgeon wanted to get me back to my natural size. So, I talked to all the nurses and told them how I felt. And I did it on purpose. I was not strong enough to make my case or have it up for discussion. I was skinny, scarred, and pretty close to being bald.

My surgeon entered the room, and I was dreading this conversation, yet it turned out to be one of the most empowering moments I have ever experienced. Not just through this whole ordeal, but in my life. He sat down, took my hands, and said, "I am on your team. You decide what you want. If you are done, you are done. We are doing it your way." I felt validated, respected, and beyond relieved. It was such a big moment for me, and I will forever be grateful for him being that sensitive and considerate to me at one of my lowest points. I really don't have the words.

I looked very different now, but I did not have the same resistance to my change as my friend did. In a weird way, the scars gave each breast a focal point and my "bald" boobs looked like they were smiling. I was, however, not as proud and thrilled about them as the gorgeous young woman I met in the waiting room was. She was really pleased about her new breasts and about herself – good for her! Some women take advantage of the situation and get their bosoms bigger than when they started, and if that is what you want – why not!

I had also calculated that by stopping refills now, I would have a month of rest. I could then have my final operation, then another month of rest, and I was just under the wire before my radiation was to begin. There is a precise and set time from when the chemo stops and radiation begins. Mine was exactly three months. My plastic surgeon reminded me that I was a cancer patient and the treatments had first priority, not the plastic surgeries themselves. My surgeon confirmed my calculation was correct, and I was in the clear. Now the reason for putting the operation ahead of the radiation is because the tissue is not as strong and resilient after radiation as healthy tissue, and you are more likely to develop complications because of it. I knew of one woman whose implants came out again. I was not going to do that to myself if I could avoid it. This, of course, does not mean it happens even if your operation is after the radiation, but it does increase the risks.

Regardless of your path, it really serves you to speak up and raise your concerns. Be willing to speak to your doctor and your nurses. They are people, just like you. Now, this doesn't mean you will get it your way. If you have questions, write them down prior to the appointment. I often showed up with a notepad. Some doctors are better equipped to deal with patients, but I found they all really wanted me to succeed and get to the other side fully cured. Your support team is extremely important, so be sure they come along as much as possible. Have a clear idea of your timeline. It can really alter your choices. You don't want to find yourself in a situation where you

say, "Had I known, my choices would have been different."
Knowledge is power, and in this situation, it can also be
life altering. You deserve and need to know.

Chapter 8

Today Is a Good Day!

*"So go ahead. Fall down. The world
looks different from the ground."*
−Oprah Winfrey

I had leaned on gratitude for a big part of my journey, but the side effects from the chemo treatments stripped me of it without me realizing it. I went through my second and final surgery and started radiation before this realization shocked me. I had been in survival-mode only. The second operation went flawlessly, and there was no pain. I was in the barn checking on the horses around noon that same day. I could now see how easily a patient could overdo her activities, especially if she received radiation prior to the surgery. I felt no pain. Actually, I felt nothing. My plastic surgeon made sure his instructions were clear before I left: *do not overdo it.* I assured my surgeon he would never, ever see me back due to any complications. I would not be overdoing anything and would follow his directions. I kept my promise to him, mainly for myself. I had already had enough, and I was absolutely committed to stay clear of any additional trips to the hospital. I was bound and determined to start radiation in a month.

My radiation oncologist was awesome. I always knew she was coming by the rhythm of her footsteps. They were sharp and precise – *tip-tap, tip-tap* – and she never dragged her heels. I was glad she was on my team. She was obviously super informed, professional, and human. Like the other doctors, she had also chosen an incredible team of nurses.

The radiation did not concern me. I had only heard good reports from other patients. The machine goes over you and then you are done. It was simple. No needles, no long days. You show up, and twenty-five minutes later, you are done. I was going to be receiving twenty-eight radiation treatments. When I met my radiation oncologist, she kind of spilled the beans. I had to have a minimum of three treatments per week. I was scheduled for five, so with a ski season approaching for my girls' school, I could skip Friday's treatment and chaperone. My oncologist was more than happy to adjust her schedule and I really appreciated that. So, I signed up as a chaperone (not surprisingly though, because of the treatments, I couldn't ski). I was glad to commit to four days a week only. It stretched the period of radiation out, which worked well for me since it was a lot to drive to Dartmouth five times a week.

The drive to Dartmouth was beautiful. It was really helpful to enjoy the beautiful countryside with open fields full of grazing cows, the Connecticut River, and beautiful traditional New England farms. I always arrived in a relaxed state of mind. I enjoyed the drive and it took my mind off the appointments ahead. I decided I would drive myself to all my radiation appointments. I was not all that strong yet, but I could get it done. Nancy had been incredibly loyal, but going through the chemo treatments was as hard on her as it was on me. She changed the Cold Caps three times an hour, and in between, prepared the next cap with a temperature gun and thick gloves to avoid frostbite. She had been completely dedicated and deserved a break. Doing these drives by myself was my way of showing her my appreciation. It gave me time to reflect on the past months alone and process them. It was healthy. There were tears that had to fall. There was the trauma of the operations, the shock of the side effects, and the knowing that I still was not done.

It had all happened so quickly. It was only a few weeks from my diagnosis to my first treatment, and those few weeks were spent preparing for the treatment plan. I had survived it all, but I had not processed it all. My plastic surgeon said to me that my body was dealing with the trauma of the operation. It took me by surprise when he said this. I had an operation, not trauma. But I realized he was right. There was so much to process, and I had just begun. The car was my space of time where things started tumbling in, and it was necessary for me to process them for long-term healing. The road was quiet, and there were a few times I needed to pull over so I could catch my breath and wipe the tears. It was a step-by-step process for me to get to the other side of the shock of the diagnosis and everything that followed. This time was still very daunting, as I was still in the middle of the treatment plan and the unknown, processing what I had been through.

There are two types of radiation, and one is more penetrating than the other. It is a very precise treatment, and I had four tiny markers tattooed on my chest. They were not supposed to hurt, but they must have hit a nerve when they put in the first marker because I jumped. But the last three markers were a breeze. I also had a body form prepared to keep me in place so the radiation would penetrate the exact same area every time. After a double mastectomy, your range of motion is compromised, and it was tough to keep my arms over my head, even when I was laying down. Every other time, I would have the normal dose and the other days, I had a bolus treatment. A wet towel was put on my chest which gave me a more concentrated dose close to my skin, as the cancer was found there.

So, the treatments started. I was surprised at how tired I got. One technician said that the daily drives were hard enough in and of themselves. He also said, "Remember, we are breaking down your body. We are attacking your cells." That was hard for me to hear. My poor body! It made sense though. It was all a war on the cells. They couldn't just pinpoint the bad ones, so my healthy cells were attacked too. All went very smoothly the first twenty radiations, and it actually went pretty quickly. I victoriously checked each day off on the schedule I was given.

After the 20th treatment all hell broke loose. The "easy" radiation turned into a challenge, and it took me right to the edge, just like chemo did. I was burned and deeply purple. Turning my head hurt, and I developed a huge blister that would crack open every time I lifted my arm. It was brutal. Every time the buzzer went off to warn me the machine was moving, I jumped in anticipation. I wasn't prepared for this severe reaction. I remember my nearest and dearest childhood friend, who was diagnosed with MS, said to me that it had to be nice knowing that there was an end to it all, to know at some point, I would be done. I mean absolutely no disrespect, but at that time, I could not see it. It was like having a burnt hand and knowing you have to stick it back in the fire "just" eight more times and then, voila, it would be over. It was absolutely overwhelming and unexpected.

I was happy to be getting treatments only four times a week and not five. If I was doing the five, I am not sure what shape I would have been in. My physical response and the mental toll surprised me and was not at all welcome. It was tough going through this last chapter in such rough shape. It finally dawned on me: I had come into chemo as a healthy person with a strong body and mind to pull from. I had reserves I could rely on and that I used for a long time – and now they were used up. When I started the radiation, I was a battered person. I had been through the wringer. I had been poisoned, sliced, and now I was being burned. It was no wonder I was giving in. The realization gave me some level of peace, but it also made those last eight treatments really tough.

I was in that radiation oncology waiting room one day, sitting as far away from the other people as I could. I was drained and simply over it. I wanted to be by myself and avoid any small talk. It was then I looked down and there was a lovely book sitting there waiting just for me. It was titled *Today Is a Good Day: A Gift of Gratitude* by Brother David Steindl-Rast. In it was a little note with well wishes. It was like finding a ray of sunshine. This blessing from a stranger gave me faith that it would all be over soon. It was such a sweet moment.

I also realized that I had not had an ounce of gratitude for a long time. I had been in survival mode, reason mode, understanding mode. I was just getting through. I kept the book. I still have it, and I will be returning it so other patients will find it. I am positive it will be picked up by the person who needs it the most so it can bring them some hope too. Though I tried my best to hide and go unnoticed that day, it didn't work. One of the many lovely volunteers was offering free massages, and just happened to be in my waiting room that day. She came and offered me a back massage. I was literally in the furthest corner, but she "found" me. She was a true blessing, and I'm glad I came to know her. The quick massage was wonderful and gave me another reason to be hopeful. Both magic moments happened on the same day. I was pretty miserable at that time, but the two wonderful events gave me back my faith that better days were on their way.

After twenty-four treatments, I simply couldn't do it anymore. I was desperate. I reached out to one of the nurses. She assured me my burned skin looked the way they expected and, as bad as it might seem, it was normal. I did finish the twenty-eight treatments, but they did back off of the bolus treatment. I could not get done soon enough. I was cooked.

Radiation was surprising. My range of motion was compromised and the effects of the treatment lasted well beyond the short treatment period. My tissue kept tightening up. I couldn't reach over my head or behind me. It felt like my tissue had been shortened and kept getting shorter. The physical therapist showed me some quick and helpful exercises, but it would take much more to get my full range of motion back. Time would be one of the biggest healers.

As great as it is to listen to others' stories, it can get you way off your path. Some women will have a hard time; some will not. We all have completely different experiences. People mean well, but all the women I spoke to had not been through a period of treatment as long as mine when they started radiation. There is value in realistic expectations. The severity of the side effects and the expectation that this would be easy were both crushing. This was not easy.

But please remember that, regardless of what others have been through, you need to keep an open mind for yourself. You might have a tougher time than the next person, but the opposite can also be true. . The unsolicited stories from other patients were not always helpful. They set me off on the wrong track of expectations. I was completely unprepared on all fronts. Be aware of the worst, yet concentrate on the positive, it will prepare you well. For better or for worse this journey is uniquely yours.

Taking just one step at a time was a really good approach for me. For me, it was one bite at a time, and that in itself could be a lot. Take your time to heal and to recover. Once you are done surviving, there will be quite a lot of healing and soul-searching to follow. Let the tears fall when they need to. So, be kind to your team, and, as always, be kind to yourself. Listen to yourself and give yourself space and time to reflect and to honor yourself. It is extremely important. Your inner voice knows what you need.

Chapter 9

Let Your Voice Be Heard

"When You Own Your Voice, You Own Your Power."
–Vocal Awareness

The radiation was finally over, but I was not done with immunotherapy. I still had another three months of that before I could put this whole part of my life behind me. But at least the trips were reduced to every three weeks and not a daily grind driving through winter blizzards on back roads. I was on the road every time there was a winter advisory to stay home. It happened to be a winter with tons and tons of snowstorms. I was on the road during Christmas break. I was in treatment on New Year's. I was looking forward to the temperature getting warmer, more daylight, and easier drives. It had been a long winter.

The immunotherapy would be completed in the spring, and I could not wait. I still had the medical port – the one that I was supposed to love, but never got comfortable with. It was uncomfortable in the vein in my neck, and after the first operation, I had to sit up to get some sort of comfort. The tubes in my neck really dug in, and the nurses were concerned as bruises developed there. When I had it put in, I had to be put under and it was relatively easy and quick. The nurses and I were chatting as I was rolled in, and during one of these conversations, I overheard them discuss the placement of the medical port. They were about to put it in my right side, the "standard" side. But I was glad I was paying attention and voiced my concern. My healthy side was the left, and the port was supposed to be inserted on that side. We were just minutes away from getting it wrong. Luckily, the nurses were quick to double check their work, and they had no problem thanking me for correcting them. The port was indeed to be placed on my left side.

The nurses were incredible. They bent over backward to accommodate us when we arrived with coolers of Cold Caps. I always had a private room. I am sure they wanted us out of the way before they tripped over all our bags and coolers, but it was still appreciated. They also knew it would be a long day for me. The hospital at that time did not endorse the Cold Cap, but the nurses knew of it and had seen Joan before. I got the strong sense they were happy to help any woman keep her hair in any way they could. It was really heart-warming. They also gave great advice and support, and I got to know some of them really well. They generously gave me warm blankets, drinks, and food – whatever I needed, they were there. They were an unbelievably wonderful group of women and men alike. They were very understanding, got the job done, and knew exactly how to carry on when they brought in the dreaded bags of chemo. They were experienced and they had the right attitude and answers. They also shed light on my situation and gave my journey a human touch. It is really helpful to have a smile, a nod, and a hug from time to time.

I was planning a trip to Denmark to celebrate a childhood friend's niece's confirmation. It was something to look forward to. I was pulling my girls out of school and we were all going together. I would see my family, be home, and eat all my favorite foods. We would be leaving less than a week after my final immunotherapy. So I had the medical port removed the second to last time, in case there were any complications. The vein in my arm could certainly handle one treatment. It seemed to be a good plan, and it worked.

The day finally came. After one-hundred and one Cold Cap changes, ten chemo drugs, twenty-eight radiation treatments, and thirty-two immunotherapy treatments, I was done. And was I ever done! I could not get out of there fast enough. When the nurse pulled that needle out of my body for the last time, I bawled. I really appreciated the hug from one of the nurses, and I really needed it.

I was so, *so* happy and relieved. I was in disbelief and also scared at the same time. I could no longer count on the treatments keeping the cancer at bay. So, now what? I felt like I was at the edge of a cliff, but mainly I was on cloud nine for the rest of the day and also shaking my head at what had just happened. I packed our bags for the trip and prepared to keep moving forward and celebrate this very big milestone. *Done!* Getting off the farm for a little bit would be good for my soul. A change of pace and scenery would take my mind off things. I was still exhausted, but it was all good. I couldn't wait to go home.

I was very much a participant in my journey. I insisted on more testing after my mammogram came back negative, I got the medical port inserted on the correct side, I spoke up when I couldn't tolerate the chemo any longer, and I got the schedule changed for the radiation treatment so I could ski with my girls. I avoided the last bolus treatments because of my burns. I got the medical port removed early. I was under the second operation after I voiced my concerns.

The clearer your idea is of what is supposed to come next and your timeline, the better off you are. You can intervene, discuss, raise concerns, and ask questions safely and without risking your best outcome. I found that the doctors and nurses were very happy to listen to me and do what they could to meet my requests when possible. I do believe I had a fabulous team. I was lucky in that I never felt I needed to question them. But if you feel you are not being heard or supported, you can always seek a second opinion, if you have time, without compromising your outcome. Whatever you do, be sure to communicate this with your medical team. You can absolutely participate in your own healing. Small changes can make your journey much easier when possible. My mom advocated for herself to get the help she needed when her treatments got off track, and my dad was a big help by being her voice. So, they were heard.

Make it as easy for yourself as you can. You have the right! Bring a loved one or a friend along. Raise your concerns. Ask all your questions. The doctors are human too, and they are here to help you, but they won't know anything's wrong unless you speak up. Talk to them and let your voice be heard. Give them the best chance of helping you get back to being you – the sooner, the better for everyone – especially you!

Chapter 10

An Ocean of Signs

"Blessings. They are everywhere.
Take time to enjoy them."
−Unknown

I have been lucky to be close to nature from childhood. I grew up in the suburbs north of Copenhagen. My love for nature kept on growing during adulthood, and it is my go-to for peace of mind. I especially have always had a very special place in my heart for the ocean – maybe because Denmark is surrounded by water. My family gathered around the TV to watch the one and only TV channel available, and on Saturday nights, it would feature the Cousteau family exploring the ocean. We were all glued to the TV. Little did I know that one day, I would be travelling the world exploring the finest reefs with a camera in hand.

There is absolutely no place like the ocean. You are immersed in wildlife when you dive, and some species will actually seek you out. You are an uninvited guest that is welcomed. You become a part of the heartbeat of the daily routine on the reef.

Imagine you are in the mountains on a cool, fall day. They are at peak fall colors with bright red, yellow, purple, and orange with splashes of green. You are weightless, flying over and in between the mountains. You fly on your back, on your side, straight ahead, and there is a herd of thirty moose cantering with you. Up ahead is a flock of geese. You fly over them. They see you and they are at ease. A bear is slowly climbing a tree, takes one quick glance at you, and goes about its business. It is relaxed and not frightened at all. This seems like fantasy, but this is very much how a diver experiences nature underwater.

I miss the close proximity to the animals, the larger-than-life experience of a pod of killer whales gliding across my view. I miss the rare moments of observing once-in-a-lifetime animal behavior. These moments with terrestrial wildlife are so fleeting. I have lived in New Hampshire now for twenty years or so, and I have seen a handful of moose and some deer. The moments are so precious and leave me longing for more time to admire and study them.

However, when I was going through my journey, I was blessed with an unusual amount of wildlife sightings. The day before I was to get my first chemo, a beautiful deer jumped right in front of me on my morning walk. It was running away, but it stopped and looked at me. Then a second one appeared. This had never happened before. Then that night, while sitting on my porch overlooking my pasture, preparing myself for the unknown, an owl flew in front of me at eye-level and across the entire pasture. I watched for a long time. It was the second owl I had ever seen on my farm. I took both of these sightings as good signs, even blessings, for the months ahead. I often saw deer driving back and forth to Dartmouth. They were the highlights of my day. They lifted my soul. One day, I opened my front door and a huge, beautiful bear was walking up the street. That was also a first. I rejoiced.

Interestingly enough, coming back home from town just last night, a beautiful deer jumped in front of my car and stopped. I had just finished Chapter 8 in this book and was emotionally drained from reliving this past year all over again. I was also sick to my stomach with self-doubt about the content of the book and the approaching deadline. After cooking dinner for my girls, I went to bed instead of working on the next chapter. But the deer inspired me not to panic. I was on track. I got the book done, and I met the strict, cast-in-stone deadline.

Nature doesn't always seem fair, but it is just. It is matter-of-fact and balanced. I have yet to find a bad sign in nature. I turn to nature all the time for both peace of mind and clarification.

Balancing of the Horses

Horses are great replacement of the ocean. Being around them keeps me balanced. We had seventeen on the farm that summer. Horses know our state of mind better than we do. As prey animals, they have to know what our intentions are. That is how they survive. They absolutely outsmart us all the time. Often when I was laying in my hammock on my porch, they would come close to be near to me. They knew I was not well and they were there to show their support. I loved hearing them breathe – it relaxed my breathing. I once even heard an animal communicator say that the horses were taking over the dolphin's role on earth. It was an interesting metaphor for me, as I was spending all my time on land when I heard this statement. True or not, they were very much concerned and were a delight to have around me. Their presence was very healing.

Take It All In

I also love angel cards and I very much turned to them during this time. When pulling them, I kept getting the Abundance card. I was to receive an abundance of support, abundance in life, and abundance in love. It was all good and it all came true – my family visiting, Nancy's support, the adoption... I also got an abundance of health. I was cured and would heal completely.

You don't have to believe in angels to fully recover. It may be too "out there" for some. But I invite you to pay attention to signs and give yourself permission to see the small messages and miracles. It can be as simple as the day I pulled into a packed parking lot – there were no spots available unless I parked really far away, and I was very tired that day. Then suddenly, a car pulled out of the absolute closest spot to the main entrance. The timing was incredible, and it was a gift. Or your signs could be the people you meet and strike up a conversation with who have the answers you have been struggling with. In my case, I talked to a woman who had her cancer recurrence ten years to the date of her first breast cancer discovery. Her words were, "Why risk it!? Why not have a double mastectomy? Make your decision as risk-free as possible." I was leaning that way any way, and hearing her say that made my decision final. I saw a flash of my girls in front of me. The deal was done, and I had no doubt about my choice. I still don't. I believe she saved me a lot of heart-ache and pain. Quite frankly, I believe she might have saved my life.

Very often, when I arrived, I felt an army of support behind me. It was all the women and men that had marched in support of a cure. It was the donors that had generously contributed to medical research and the thousands of people showing up on behalf of their loved ones. I felt a massive body of energy walking behind me, and they were there to push me through the door every time.

I could feel them so strongly, I could almost see their faces. They were real! It was an experience unlike any other, one that happily surprised me. It still gives me goosebumps.

But it was not just the people that had gone before me or supported the cause – it was also the angelic support from the nurses and the volunteers. We were blessed with incredible volunteers that would fuss over us. I was given Reiki almost every time I had my infusions. There was a lovely lady, a breast cancer survivor herself, who was healing us as she was healing herself. I also met a woman who was going around and offering free chair massages. When she wasn't doing that, she went around with lavender/thyme massage oil specially ordered from an organic farm in North Carolina and rubbed our feet. We connected and came to find out we both had adopted African American children, so there was an instant bond. A coincidence? I don't think so. She was so wonderful and put my last infusion on her calendar so she could be there with me to celebrate. And we did. She was right there, and as usual, the relaxing effect of her foot rub made a huge difference not only in how I felt, but also in the effectiveness of the treatments.

For you, a song might inspire you, or a call from a friend you haven't heard from in years. Maybe it's a fleeting thought, a commercial on TV, or a bird flying by. I hold on to all of these as messages of encouragement, lessons to be learned, things to pay attention to, glimpses of hope, and hugs from the universe. Whatever you believe in,

I hope you allow yourself to tune in if you haven't already. You might be more prepared to receive the signs meant for you.

I found this to be true as I was uneasy, worried, and a bit more vulnerable than normal – my guards were down. For the outside world, this might seem a bit crazy, and it can be a very personal part of your journey. Stick with it. Use whatever it is that helps you and lifts your soul! There is support all around you from the most surprising sources. I held on to every sign, and paid attention to and embraced all the blessings that were given to you. All the coincidences are there to help you and show up when you need them the most. Accept the help from others and embrace the support that is being offered to you. Do it wholeheartedly. It will help you and might even save your life.

Chapter 11

Your Pals

*"Once women find sisterhood, there
is nothing stronger."*
–Zoe Kravitz

No matter how hard people try or how well inten-
tioned people are, nobody (including me and you)
can truly relate to somebody or a situation until they
have been in it. It doesn't matter what it is – I will never
know what my mom goes through on a daily basis with
her fibromyalgia or what my friend who got diagnosed
with MS goes through. Because of this, your surviving
sisters are invaluable.

I was very naive going into this, even though I had
been through a lot with my mom. I had way too many
assumptions that were wrong. I had no idea how many

faces of breast cancer there were. When I made my decision on the double mastectomy, I simply couldn't fathom how anyone would make any decision other than the one I did. I almost thought these other women were careless.

But so many factors influence your decisions. Are you in a relationship? Do you have kids? Did other members of your family have it or not? I was in my fifties, not my twenties. Life looks very different as each decade passes. The journey is humbling and I was quick to drop my judgment, especially after joining the PALS program. It became more and more obvious that there were tons of options and just as many different situations. My choice became the obvious and only choice for me. The urgency in my situation created clarity and was very helpful, but each woman and circumstance are different. Joining this group completely cemented this understanding.

By being around other women and listening to their stories, I also got really informed. You will get full understanding and no judgment from them when you are a no-show to a planned event or get-together. Chemo brain is absolutely real and can last a while. I once had an appointment with a survivor, but she never showed and never acknowledged that she forgot. The appointment most likely never made it on her calendar and poof – it evaporated into thin air. I knew exactly what happened and I never brought it up. It's just part of the deal. I know I have done the same – I just don't remember it! The great part of survivors is that you can have a great sense of humor around them. They know what you are going through and they know when to laugh and when to put the brakes on. You are all on the inside, unlike all the healthy folks who are tip-toeing around unsure how best to act around you. That in itself can be exhausting when you have to assure someone that it is okay to talk about it.

To Tell or Not to Tell

It wasn't my choice to keep my cancer secret; I did it out of necessity and out of fear that my hopefully-soon-to-be adopted girl would be taken away if the DCYF found out about the state of my health. I couldn't afford to take the risk. It was worth it and absolutely had some benefits. Cancer was not the main topic of all conversations in my life. It kept a sense of normalcy. It wasn't until all my treatments were over and the adoption had happened that I posted the good news on Facebook. But I also knew some women who wanted their friends and family to know. Telling their story was healing for them. The attention is nice and the support can be great. It is heartwarming to hear from old friends that are now reaching out to you, or hearing from other survivors and having them cheer you on.

When my diagnosis became public, there was a lot of concern from lots of people. It was so appreciated and the positive vibes were very much part of my healing. I truly know this now. But just be aware it can also be a lot to answer everyone's questions. Some want continuous updates, and at times, this is a lot to handle. Ask them to connect with you through a family member. You must conserve energy for your healing and not answer questions or give updates to the masses.

You might find some people can't be around you. It might trigger them if they themselves went through it themselves or with a loved one. I know I had a couple situations I had to pull back from because I knew they would trigger me. I have finally learned to protect myself. It is a must!

To Know or Not to Know

Some of us are information gatherers and some of us are not. I was supposed to get tested for the cancer gene. It is required by law that I meet in person with the doctor who can explain the pros and cons and make sure I fully understand all the ramifications based upon the results from the test. My appointment was scheduled between my fourth and fifth chemo treatments and I simply did not have another drive or appointment in me. I had to reserve my energy for the more urgent requirements.

So, I canceled. I was going to have the double mastectomy anyway, which was the main purpose for the test. I could have done it now, but I have decided against it; I really don't want to know. I have managed to keep my fears at bay and I don't want to rock the boat by feeling something is wrong or being on alert all the time. I passed on seeing my MRI, where the issue on my right side lit up like a Christmas tree. To this day, it would scare me to see it. It was too much reality, too scary and it would not serve me in any way.

But for some, the more informed they have, the better. It is a very personal choice. I spoke with one women and she absolutely compiled every bit of information she could find on cancer and her diagnosis. She read everything and was completely informed. She felt it was the part of her journey she had control over and she dwelled in this control. It was her way to fully participate in her own healing. Some find comfort in the facts. It is something worth considering. Do you really want to know? The information could scare you. I met another woman who had googled what kind of a CAT scan she would have. It made her absolutely terrified. Her teeth were chattering while she waited. She absolutely regretted knowing too much. I really liked my pace. I took it one appointment at a time and it felt very manageable. I was going through this huge ordeal one bit at a time, and for me, that was the way to go.

When the last treatment is over with, you will most likely be very elated and then terrified. It happened to my mom and it happened to me. So, now what? There are well over 250,000 women diagnosed with cancer annually. Yet, it can be hard to find a support group. However, I was so lucky to be included in the PALS program. It is a twelve-week physical rehabilitation program developed specifically for breast cancer survivors. It was started by a young woman, Erin Buck, who had lots of challenging times in her own life, none of which were cancer! She was and is fabulous, and I only hold gratitude in my heart for her.

She worked closely with a physician to develop this program. I later found out that it happened to be my surgeon! I gladly joined the twelve-week PALS program during the summer, and we sat down and introduced ourselves. I was really down emotionally and started to bawl. One woman simply put her hand on mine. It was a touch of understanding and compassion that could only come from another survivor. The gesture meant the world to me.

I was still undergoing immunotherapy, so I had to miss some of the workouts. We were given worksheets to keep track of our progress. We were only allowed to lift one-pound weights. One pound! It was a dose of reality – talk about starting over! During the first twelve weeks, I was in a very frail mental and physical condition and couldn't benefit as much as the other participants did. But I did learn some of the participants were accepted into the program though their diagnoses and treatments happened years ago. The effects were still very real for them and the emotional impact and support from the groups was still very beneficial to these women, regardless of the years that had passed! They were welcomed, honored, and justified. You don't have to be a super survivor to have your story be heard. Most aren't, but the comfort of being in a group with like-minded women is second to none. This group in particular were all active participants in their own recovery and invested in their future by showing up for the workouts the best they could. They all wanted to get better and believed they would. They did everything they could to give themselves the best shot at life and make the best out of every day.

We started again the following fall in the Bridge Program, also led by Erin, and we were really happy to see each other. This was also a twelve-week program that included a talk from Dr. Laleh. Once the twelve weeks were over, we took a break and were invited to a "graduation" in January. There, we were gathered to paint a canvas. I had not seen these women for months and it was like coming home. I realized then how essential my interactions with them were. These were my partners in survival.

I was also accepted into a weekend program, Casting for Recovery – it is a great program and it is in most of the fifty states. I was going fly-fishing! How fun! It is invitation only – in other words, your medical team needs to confirm you are a candidate. I would absolutely find out if this program is available in your state. Talk to your oncologist and nurse (it was my nurse that got me in). It was an absolutely delightful experience. I had chemo brain for sure, and when I entered the foyer, a welcome committee was sitting, and I saw a familiar face. I couldn't place her, but I just knew I was happy to see her. I eventually realized it was the nurse with healthy curls: Stacy. It was *so* good to see her, and the depth of her dedication to the well-being of her patients and other women became very real. She was volunteering and spending time away from her family to be with us. I was beyond lucky, blessed, and couldn't have been happier. Stacy was actually the one who accepted my application for the fly fishing program.

It was a great weekend. The New Hampshire women were quite ready for this special opportunity. It was really lovely, and in our first evening meeting, our conversations were very honest and open. There was one particular woman who I keep in touch with on a very irregular basis. I absolutely adored her. She was very funny and up front. She also made a great comment: she felt sicker during this weekend retreat than going to the hospital, because the cancer was talked about so much. I could relate. I very carefully measured what served me and what did not. I mean no disrespect to anybody when I say I don't consider myself a survivor. I simply never considered not surviving. It was not an option. I got why she felt the same way. However, I found it very helpful, and the women were there to enjoy, learn, and participate. They had the right attitude. There is simply a built-in knowing and understanding of where the women in the group were at depending on what they were going through. Some had just had chemo. One was celebrating ten healthy years. Interestingly enough, there is a very relaxed attitude towards breast cancer. One woman had a preventive mastectomy and she still got cancer. She also got cured, so it was all good.

I can't imagine not having my Surviving Sisters, but as with all situations, you have to judge what helps and works for you. Most likely whatever you choose is good, but it might not be. Stay true to yourself. Dive in if it serves you and bail if it doesn't. It is your journey and you need to make the choices that heal you. This is not the time to consider others' feelings or if you offend anybody. You simply have the right to fully heal.

Chapter 12

Have What You Want!

*"If you correct your mind the rest of
your life will fall into place."*
–Lao Tzu

I have been blessed to spend seventeen falls diving during the prime season in the Solomon Islands. It is truly my home away from home. I love the boat, the sweet smells from the islands, the beautiful people, the dug-out canoes. Kokoana Passage is one of my favorite dive sites. It's one of the passages between the islets that creates the barrier between the Pacific Ocean and Marovo Lagoon, the largest lagoon in the world. The best diving is when the tides are coming into the lagoon, as it brings the clear ocean water. When its current runs out, visibility drops as it fills with murky lagoon water. There was a sense of adventure being so close to the edge of the vast ocean with no land in sight for hundreds of miles. The currents can be strong, but it is the very current that is the life source for the reef and the ocean.

There was one particular dive I still remember at Kokoana Passage. We had just visited one of the villages to buy their produce, baskets, and woodcarvings. It was midafternoon and there was still enough daylight to be able to photograph, yet it was just late enough the sun rays were starting to have that golden, magical light. There was a softness to the light, yet the current was ripping into the lagoon with clear ocean water. With my camera housing in hand, I was ready to go. I had never ever seen conditions this perfect. I was awestruck, slack-jawed, and amazed. After a while, I gave up taking pictures. There are moments that just need to be experienced.

This was a blessing. The current carried me as I watched one sea fan more beautiful than the next. The sun rays beamed through the surface, and the wall was alive with schooling fish feasting on the plankton. What a sight. After years of diving here, I had never seen it this perfect. It was a moment with conditions of a lifetime. I didn't want this dive to end, and when I reached the end of the dive site, I turned around, swam against the current, glided back, and did the dive all over again. It was truly magic! When I got back to the boat, I was thrilled. Surely my guests would have had a fantastic time as well! Then one of our divers said, "I don't get it. Why did we come here – it is just a big wall of sea fans!"

We can be in the exact same place, yet have a completely different experience. We can have an ocean full of blessings yet have completely opposite experiences. I was glad I saw the moment and all the beauty in it.

I do believe our cancer journeys are a matter of perspective, just like the dive at Kokoana Passage. We were there at the same place at the same time, and yet we had two completely different experiences. We do have a choice on how we get through the day. Being in a positive state of mind is simply a healthy state of mind.

Gratitude is an absolute must for living the best life you can ever live. The deeper and longer I dive into the positive effects of a positive mindset on health, as well as the power of visualizing a future, the clearer it becomes that it's working. Gratitude absolutely played a big part in my outcome. I do daily exercises now, but even before I started doing daily work, I already began taking inventory of all I had already manifested.

Going all the way back to my childhood, I dreamt of scuba diving, but the rhythm of a Danish life was laid out for me: grade school, high school, travel for a year or two before starting a higher education, find an apartment or buy a house with somebody. Underwater photography was not on anybody's radar. When I worked in California for a year, I got my scuba diving certification, and I was given a coffee table book. I simply couldn't look through the pages, as I was finishing up my stay overseas and was starting to think of going home to start my education. To make a long story short, life took a big turn, and almost thirty years and thousands and thousands of images and dives later, I realize I very much manifested my dreams of traveling, not knowing it would take me all over the world to the most remote dive sites like the Galapagos Islands, Cocos Island, Papua New Guinea, Solomon Islands, Vanuatu, Australia, Egypt, and Indonesia, or that I would become an award-winning underwater photographer.

There are many ways we are taught how to manifest the life of our dreams. It can be through repetition of your wishes by saying them, writing them down, visualizing them in your mind and connecting to how you feel when you have accomplished your goals, or creating a vision board. I use most of these techniques myself. But I have also found that a deeply grounded yearning also works, and it only takes one sentence.

One day, while going through some old paperwork, I came across an address to an adoption website. I wrote that in the back of my address book where I knew for sure no one would ever see it. I was in a marriage where there was no room or time for children. We traveled half the year and our livelihood was traveling. We saw the obvious signs of over-population. I could make sense of my situation, but my heart truly never felt at peace. Was my purpose to be a mom or was it my deeply inner wish that couldn't be silenced? I don't know.

When I got out of that marriage, I became a licensed foster parent. When I saw a tiny picture of my first daughter, I would have adopted her right then and there. It took about one year before the adoption was finalized. Once she was settled, we started talking about a sister. So, I said I would extend my foster parent license and would adopt. I wrote down my criteria: "I want an African American or bi-racial girl three to six years of age, and I want her to be available for immediate adoption." That is a lot to ask for. The African American population in New Hampshire is one percent. But then I got the call when I was in Denmark, and the day after returning, I went to meet my soon-to-be daughter, and became a mom for the second time months later.

The day I realized I had manifested this deep wish of becoming a mom, I had to sit down. There was no way in my wildest dreams that I thought, when I wrote the wish down, the pieces in my life could ever be put in an order for this to happen. There was no way. I might as well have written down that I wanted to walk on the moon when I wrote down that adoption site years earlier. That is why I know now that big, bold, and beautiful ideas and dreams are really possible. I aim high now. However, I consider becoming a mom the manifestation of a lifetime.

Another of my visions was a waterfront property. I had it written down as part of my manifestation wish list. It was another impossible dream. Even fixer uppers were more than we wanted to spend, knowing the cost of bringing it up to livable standards. The one year anniversary of my diagnosis, I "accidentally" came across a super-cute seasonal cottage with a deck perched on the water's edge, just twenty-five minutes from our farm. The price was beyond belief and well in our budget. I had just sold some other real estate, and the pieces came together perfectly. The cottage was ours less than a month after I found it. Now, we sit on our deck perched over the thirty-five acres of water and watch the resident turtles swimming around. Last summer, we enjoyed a pair of loons. We enjoy the sunsets.

I am now working in my newly remodeled office. It is absolutely perfect, and another item off my wish list. I had no idea I would ever have an office this wonderful. I love leaning back in my office chair and see the pasture and the horses roaming in it.

I always gave thanks to my healthy body as part of my daily gratitude journal. Some would argue that it didn't work, but I say it absolutely did. I was not in good health at the time, but by being my own advocate, I was diagnosed in time for a textbook-perfect outcome. With that, I am keener now more than ever to move forward into manifestation and take more control of my own destiny. Do I ever get scared? Sometimes fear does creep up on me, but the feeling doesn't stick around for long. I have built a mental muscle that helps me move away from fear. Fear is like praying for something you don't want. I still do exercises when my mind can stay positive. One of my frequent angel cards reads: "Focusing on what you want is like putting your hands on the steering wheel of your life." Now that doesn't mean it won't be a winding road, but it does give a lot of hope and reasons to be optimistic. And I am.

I look into the future. I visualize picking up my grand-children from school. My oldest is thirteen and my youngest is eight now, so I am visualizing that far into the future. It is intentional. I demand a full, long, happy, prosperous, peaceful, carefree, fulfilled, and healthy life. I have become very aware of my language, thoughts, and perspective. It is very powerful.

I suggest, even if you are not really resonating with this idea of manifestation, you take a look at your own life. There might be some things you already focused on that came into fruition. You might surprise yourself with how much you've already done. Sometimes it can be the neg-ative things you focused on. A quick example is a wish to be cancer-free. Being perfectly healthy is a better option as you focus on health, not sickness. Or instead of wishing to be mortgage-free, a better choice would be, "owning in full." The intentions are the same, but one sends out negative vibes and the other sends positive vibes. Go for the good vibes!

It takes discipline and effort to build a mental muscle that will build your belief and desires. Positive thinking will influence your well-being, no matter what. You don't have to be a superstar at this. If you begin right now, you will better your life.

Fear is part of this as well. You will experience a full range of emotions in your journey, and you can help yourself move past them. I have practiced and am getting better at this all the time. I am not perfect, but I am trying my best. My wish for you is that you find peace of mind and believe that you have a long and healthy life ahead of you. Imagine, what you will do? Imagine the life of your dreams – anything you want. What would your perfect day be like? Where would you be? What would you be doing? Who would you be with? Say it out loud, if that is what it takes to override the fear. Dive in and visualize your best life ever, even if it is just in your dreams for now. Chant it in your car. Write them down a thousand times. Write down all your dreams and write them as if you are already living them and they have already materialized. Keep going until you can feel, believe, and see yourself doing all you would love to. There is a great saying you might have heard: "What would you do if you could not fail?" or even better, "What would you do if your success was absolutely guaranteed?" What would you do? Make your dreams big and bold. Now go live them.

Chapter 13

The Pink Lemon

"The biggest adventure you can take
is living the life of your dreams."
−Oprah Winfrey

So, life handed you a lemon. You could make lemon-
ade, but there was no way I was going to spend any
more time than necessary with this lemon, and I certainly
wasn't going to add sugar. Somewhere, I read that freezing
the lemon and throwing it back where it came from was
another alternative. This is the road and metaphor that
worked for me. I had a good attitude through most of this
journey, but I never embraced my situation. I never would
have been proud of my bald head, like some admirable and
brave women are. I look at them in awe and salute them,
but that was not me. I focused on getting through this as
quickly as possible.

It is surprising how many faces breast cancer has. When I joined the PALS program, I learned from the other women there that cancer showed up in so many ways. Some of the women had it quite easy, and some had much longer treatments (like I did). Well, still do – I will continue to take my daily estrogen repression pill for seven years, as my cancer was fueled by estrogen. But regardless of the stage or the type of treatment we had, we had all been affected by our diagnoses. That's a big deal. It was heartwarming to see how much we needed each other and how we all advanced and strengthened our bodies and our hope and outlook for the future together.

This is uniquely your journey. I give you permission to make the choices you want that suit you best and resonate with you. There will be choices you make that might not make any sense to the people around you. They may not agree with them or they might question you. When you make your decisions, especially about an operation or lack thereof, ask yourself, "How will I feel if, after this, the cancer returns?" The chances of it returning and the risks should be understood and discussed with your doctors. Make a pros and cons list to help get all the facts and considerations in one place.

So much has been done in the breast cancer field, and we have come so far. "No one dies of breast cancer" was what I thought my surgeon said to me. This is not a true statement. She actually said something along the lines of, "Cancer is extremely curable." We still have a cloud hanging over us when we are diagnosed with breast cancer, but for most, it's a much lighter cloud now, and this needs to be recognized. We have so much to be optimistic about. Some treatments are becoming almost routine when detected early. It is very encouraging.

Looking back, I realize I was in denial – a lot. I didn't entertain all the "what-ifs." I also heard a lot of the information incorrectly. I wonder if this was my brain's way of shutting off when I couldn't process any more information. Maybe it is a survival mechanism that sets in before you get paralyzed with fear.

There is so much more I could learn and know about breast cancer. I got through mostly all my appointments. I joined the PALS programs and continued in the Bridge program. The day the Bridge program ended, I signed up to write this book. I have put so much of my breast cancer journey behind me, but it is also very fresh with me still. As every day passes, I get better. I believe I am almost back to normal, but I still pay attention to anything my body tells me. Sleep is a must for me, so I am protective of it. I also make sure I don't commit myself to more than I can handle on my schedule. I have been in several situations where other friends' health and other situations have been tasking and more than I could handle. So, I will remove myself from that situation, if necessary. It's not that I am not sympathetic, but it's because I have to protect my health first and foremost.

Traveling around the world diving the world's most fabulous dive sites has been a journey of excitement, awe, and disbelief – it is truly a world of wonder. But it was my journey back to health that gave my life depth. I am now enriched with a deeper understanding of life. I now know what physical pain feels like. I can appreciate the freedom a child feels when she is out of the wheelchair and on a horse for the first time, especially after I rode my mare and it was hard for me to breath. I know what it means to be tired all the way to my core and what it means to have support. It is very healing for the soul to surrender and experience the people around you who are able to catch you. I can now relate to and help others. I know what it means to be cured! It is my gold medal in life.

For me, this diagnosis was the ultimate wake-up call. As I keep moving forward, I also slide back into old habits. It is a good sign, I suppose, that life is getting back to normal. But I try to make sure I don't repeat the stress and other emotions that were part of the reason I got sick in the first place. I push through the doubts and fears standing in the way of my dreams, like writing this book. I won't allow emotions or wishes to get bottled up inside of me. I communicate better and no longer put myself on the back burner. This is not a selfless act, but it is absolutely a necessity for a healthy future. I am staying healthy. Period. This is a choice and I am acting on it. I do not keep track of any of the big milestone dates. As far as I am concerned, this chapter of my life is behind me. The less time I spend revisiting it, the better it is for me.

I hope you will envision yourself as a healthy woman who is taking charge of your life and honoring yourself by putting yourself first, not just for you, but for your loved ones. Ask all questions you want, stand tall, and believe you will be stronger than ever. Eat healthier, trust in your intuition and all the signs that are sent to you, or whatever helps you, even if and when this is not embraced by your loved ones. I hope you will feel the helpful spirit of millions of people that truly want your full recovery to be an absolute success.

"Someday" is today. The future has arrived. Today is the day to act on your dreams, whatever they are. Your dreams are perfect, even if they might not follow what is expected of you. Unclutter your life, spend more time with your family and friends, and find peace of mind and simplicity. Go on a trip. Change your career, start a business, or get out of the rat race. Get a degree. Learn to sing, or act on a lifelong dream. Take up belly-dancing! Move to the country, or move to the city. Live a year overseas. Volunteer. Write a book! Whatever your dreams are, they are perfect. If you have any old dream still in your heart, now is the time to act on it and see it come true.

Remember, there is no expiration date on a dream, and it is never too old. Bring it to life. Inspire the world around you. Show us all how much you can shine. Create the life you dream of. You deserve it, and it is where you belong! Make it healthy, make it exciting, make it deeply fulfilling, make it fun, make it bold, and most of all, make it last far, *far* into the future!

Acknowledgments

There is no way you can get through this journey by yourself and still have the best outcome possible. I have many to thank for helping me through my journey. These wonderful people include:

My mom and dad, who were great support and traveled from Denmark twice to be with me during the hardest of times.

My brother, Per, who came over as well. There is nothing like family and a sense of home and humor.

Deb and Willi for your daily calls.

Charlie for being our go to guy and for always being there for us.

Åse og Frank for always being there.

Mette Lærke for always calling me, even when you weren't feeling well!

Mike and Carol Anne for being awesome and supportive friends.

Claire, Don, and Meghan for your home-cooked meals and support.

Ginny and John for always checking in on me.

Holly and Jay helping out with the girls.

Helle and Per for checking in on me.

Tammy for being a great farm-sitter.

Chub for helping and making summer vacation fun for the kids.

Carolina and Anna for grabbing Tavi for several overnights.

Janine for having the girls for a weekend.

Irene for letting my family use your pool.

To Barbara and Lori for being great friends and sending me the charm loaded with good vibes.

All the women I spoke with along the way who helped me.

Everyone who reached out to help.

Shirley Sullivan and everyone at Farms and Barns for your patience and support.

Joan and her volunteers with Fat Hat Clothing Company for providing Cold Caps.

My entire medical team and Dartmouth staff.

All the wonderful musicians, Reiki therapists, and massage therapists who volunteered at Dartmouth.

Erin Buck, the creator of the PALS and bridge program, and Dr. Laleh, for all your valuable nutritional information.

All my wonderful PALS and Bridge ladies.

The Casting For Recovery group for a fabulous weekend.

Joanne – what would we have done without you? Thank you for all the home-cooked meals, even the ones I couldn't eat! You were our angel.

Angela Lauria and the incredible team I worked with at the Author Incubator. Ramses Rodriquez for being there. Emily Tuttle and Moriah Richard, you are both beyond words wonderful.

My dog Jack for never leaving my side and keeping me company either by my bed or on it. And to Mille, Bongo, Maddie and Gracie and all the beautiful horses.

Tavari and Sierra for patiently putting up with me during this long haul.

And last but not least, Nancy for always being there wholeheartedly. I can never thank you enough!

Thank You

Hello, beautiful reader,

Thank you so much for reading *Live Well beyond Breast Cancer*. I sincerely hope it inspired you or somehow helped you in a small or big way. I know hearing other women's stories made a world of a difference to me.

I am developing a program for women just like you who want to get through this with the best possible outcome. Does this sound familiar? If so, please feel free to email me at dedawilms@gmail.com, private message me on my Facebook page, or visit my web-site www.pinklemoncoaching.com.

I look forward to hearing from you. You are appreciated and worthy of support, love, and a full recovery.

With an ocean of gratitude and love,
Birgitte

About the Author

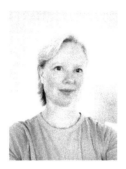

Native to Denmark, Birgitte Wilms is an award-winning underwater photographer and best-selling author. She has been inducted into the Women's Divers Hall of fame and is now a stage-4 breast cancer survivor.

Her underwater images are published internationally in prestige magazines like LIFE, National Geographic etc. Her images are also displayed in the Smithsonian Museum in Washington, DC. She is a co-author of the award-winning book, *In a Sea of Dreams.* She is currently working on a children's book series and an online children's educational series, along with other children's products featuring the oceans and its inhabitants.

Birgitte is now using her decades of experience hosting international underwater photo expeditions, her people skills, and her own journey through cancer and back to health to offer support and guide other women, individuals, or groups in their unique journey. She also hosts retreats for women on her 260 acre farm – a perfect place for rejuvenation with private trails by the river, mountain views, and privacy. Birgitte is also a mother of two, land photographer, horseback rider, a real estate agent, an Airbnb superhost and an avid gardener. Birgitte lives in Central New Hampshire with her family, dogs, and horses.

CPSIA information can be obtained
at www.ICGtesting.com
Printed in the USA
JSHW021617221220
10505JS00006B/175

9 781953 153234